Learn to Sign

WITH YOUR

BABY

50 ESSENTIAL ASL SIGNS
TO HELP YOUR CHILD COMMUNICATE THEIR
NEEDS, WANTS, AND FEELINGS

Cecilia S. Grugan

Illustrated by Brittany Castle

ZEITGEIST • NEW YORK

For Mama and Papa,
who ensured my
access to language

ISBN: 9780593435625

Ebook ISBN: 9780593435632

Author photograph © by Capitol Hill Portraits: Timothy Devine
Illustrator photograph © by YoungMi Mannino 2022

Illustrations by Brittany Castle

Design by Aimee Fleck and Katy Brown

Actor for ASL videos: Joseph "Joey" Antonio

Printed in the United States of America

3 5 7 9 10 8 6 4 2

First Edition

Contents

~~~~~

Introduction

Welcome to my world of sign language with babies! In my world, the morning begins with a bottle for my baby, some tea for me, and the sign for "Drink." I log on to my computer, signing "Computer," and take a peek at my telework schedule for the day. Next comes a diaper change and choosing a daytime outfit for my baby, accompanied by the sign for "Change." I bounce them on my knee and sign "Work." With one hand, I type a few email responses for my daytime job. A brisk walk with the stroller follows my work routine, and I sign "Stroller" before my baby dozes off. When my baby wakes up, I log off my computer and get right to making dinner, signing "Food" to my baby. After dinner, it's cleanup time—and my baby's favorite time of day, which I initiate with the sign for "Bath."

Just like any other parent or caregiver (I'll be using "parent" and "caregiver" interchangeably), I'm juggling multiple responsibilities while caring for a baby on a daily basis. *Unlike* many other caregivers, whatever it is I'm doing, I use sign language with my baby. Thanks to sign language, I'm able to communicate with my baby in comprehensible ways, and we are forming a unique connection.

I was a baby myself—just 15 months old—when my parents learned that I'm deaf. The first thing my hearing parents did was buy *The Joy of Signing*. They immediately exposed me to sign language at home, coupled with spoken language. However, when I came of age, I went to school and participated in sports and social events populated primarily by hearing peers. It wasn't until I turned 18 and attended a college with a large Deaf population that my world of sign language opened up again.

After graduation, I found myself back in the hearing world until I met my life partner, Maya, who is also Deaf. Like many other couples, Maya and I wanted to raise a family together. Now, as parents, we want what all parents want. We want to connect with our child. We want them to comprehend the language we use, and we want to understand their efforts to communicate with us. So, sign language it is!

But sign language isn't just for the Deaf. Anybody can learn sign language for any reason. In this book, we'll explore sign language as it relates to the special baby in your life. With a bit of enthusiasm and a willingness to learn, hearing parents can communicate with their children using sign language, too. In this book, I'll offer suggestions and guidance to help you make decisions relevant to using sign language in your unique situation. As you read on, you'll discover how special it can be to sign with your baby. One of the greatest benefits that signing caregivers witness is their child's ability to express themself sooner than if the caregivers use only spoken language with them. By including sign language as a part of your baby's upbringing, you will maximize your chances of a deeper, language-rich connection.

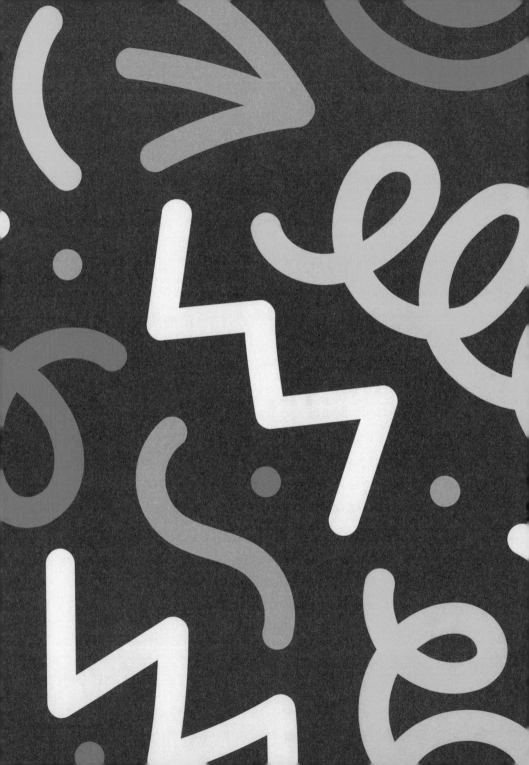

CHAPTER 1

Signing for Babies 101

Congratulations for initiating what will be a delightfully rewarding endeavor for you and your child. This chapter will provide you with the information you need to start signing with your baby. I'll answer questions like "Why sign with my baby?" and "How do I learn and teach sign language to my baby?" You'll be excited to discover that using sign language with even the youngest child is totally possible!

Welcome to ASL for Babies!

American Sign Language (ASL) is an official language (used just in the United States). It includes its own linguistic properties of grammar and syntax, and it's important to acknowledge that ASL does not follow English structure, but it's easy to learn because you can start communicating with just one word.

Signing with babies is an increasingly popular approach to communicating with them, and ASL is being used well beyond the Deaf community. Parents and caregivers have come to realize that signing with a baby is monumental and beneficial because signing with a baby, even as a newborn, can increase the likelihood of comprehensible communication before verbal development. This means you may be communicating with your child earlier than you had imagined—how exciting would that be?

While this book will share nuances about the Deaf culture and ASL, I will not focus on complete sentences using ASL grammar and syntax. Rather, this book is meant to teach simple vocabulary words. Each of the words you'll be learning is accompanied by two tips in any of the following categories:

Memory Hack: A way to remember how a sign is done; typically a visual

Helping Hand: A tip for helping your baby do a sign or a suggestion for how to use a sign contextually

Watch for This! Something to be aware of, such as how your baby might make early attempts at a particular sign

Have Fun! How to integrate a sign into opportunities for play

One important thing to note before we continue: The signs in this book are not made up or modified. The signs you will learn and use with your baby are the same signs that members of all ages in the Deaf community use. Finally, remember that while an ASL book can provide instructions for forming signs, it's highly encouraged that you continue learning ASL face-to-face with a Deaf instructor, either virtually or in person, after you've gone through this book (see the resources section, page 150).

Videos for Every Sign

ASL is a visual language and is not really designed to be described in writing. For ease of learning, we have included videos accessible through this QR code (along with illustrations) for all the vocabulary words covered in this book so you can see exactly how they are signed.

You can also access the videos at **signwithyourbaby.zeitgeistpublishing.com**.

Why Sign with Your Baby?

There are many benefits of signing with your baby:

- **Signing replaces frustration, crying, and meltdowns with understanding and connection.** Imagine a baby signing what they need or want, when all they could do before was cry. Sign language is a tool that a baby can use to express themself before they can vocalize words. With a signing baby, a caregiver can respond more effectively.

- **A baby's ability to express themself will increase their sense of self.** One of the most attainable ways to enhance a baby's ability to communicate is with sign language. If a baby knows the signs, they can tell you if they want their favorite stuffed animal or if they are all done with the mango purée. When babies feel understood, they become empowered to further express themselves.

- **You are introducing a diverse world and its meaningful differences.** By using sign language with your baby, you are opening the door to another language, culture, and community. You are providing your baby with a foundation of acceptance and understanding of others' differences.
- **You and your baby will form a stronger and more significant connection.** For a caregiver, there is an innate desire to connect with your baby. Such a bond can be created by providing physical affection, nourishment, and a warm space to sleep. Additionally, if you sign with your baby, they will develop a sense of belonging as a result of effective communication, leading to a stronger bond.
- **Sign language is a versatile language.** You can use sign language to adapt to a variety of environments for ease of communication. For example, you can communicate in total silence so as not to disrupt a work meeting or a religious service. You can sign to your baby while listening to someone on the phone. You can use sign language to communicate underwater. You can even sign over the roar of an airplane!

How to Get Started

Aha! You may have turned right to this section because you're eager to jump right in. You're excited to know how to use sign language with your baby. That's understandable! One of the most popular questions caregivers ask about using sign language with their baby is, "Where do I begin?"

This section will give you the basics for how to start using ASL with your baby. It will also help you set realistic expectations for how to navigate this journey.

At first, you may wonder if you're juggling too much, especially with a baby under your care. Good news: Learning sign language with your baby can happen as you go about your daily routine! You don't need to read this book in one sitting. Rather, you can sneak in a quick moment to learn and practice a particular sign. A great place to begin is with the starter signs in chapter 2 (page 25). These signs include useful words such as "Eat" (page 28) and "All Done" (page 32). You may want to start elsewhere—that's okay, too! For instance, you may wonder what sign you could use for a bedtime routine. Refer to chapter 5 (page 93) for sleeping and rising signs. Once you've acquired the sign for, say, "Goodnight" (page 96), you can give it a try the same evening. When you feel comfortable using one sign with your baby, move on to the next.

Before you get started, I have more good news to share with you. You're probably already using your hands to communicate with your baby. There are some universal gestures you may be familiar with and even currently use with your baby:

- Waving to someone in greeting or farewell is you signing "Hello" or "Goodbye."
- Shaking your head from side to side or nodding up and down a couple of times is one way of signing "No" and "Yes," respectively.

- Extending your arm and wagging your wrist back and forth toward yourself is gesturing "Come here."
- If you're saying "Shh" or "Be quiet," there's a good chance you're also signing it by putting your index finger across the surface of your puckered lips.

It's important to keep in mind that the above-mentioned are universal gestures and not unique to American Sign Language. Nevertheless, you're well on your way to using your hands to sign with your baby!

When to Start and with What Signs

Another popular question caregivers ask is, "When do I begin?" Here's a simple answer: There is no one right age. Also, it is never too late to begin. When your baby is born, you can begin the moment they arrive earthside! *But what would I sign to my newborn?* you may wonder. Since your baby starts to feed from the moment they're born, you can start signing words like "Milk" (page 26) or "Bottle" (page 72) right away. Additionally, you can sign "Change" (page 116) and "Diaper" (page 114) early on, too. Your newborn may not pick up on these signs; however, every child is different and acquires language in their own time and at their own pace. Some pick up language much sooner than anticipated. Essentially, you are signing to your baby whenever you can because they may pick up on a sign at any time! No matter when you begin signing with your child, you are building a strong foundation in communicating via sign language.

Teaching Yourself and Your Baby to Sign

You may have some questions about teaching and learning sign language:

- **How do I find time to learn sign language?** You can learn in snippets that won't take more than a few minutes of your time. While you're waiting for your coffee order, practice learning how to sign "Drink" (page 70). While you're waiting for your dinner to finish cooking in the oven, learn how to sign "Eat" (page 28). With a few quiet moments in the evening, you can learn how to sign "Goodnight" and "Bed" (page 98).

- **How do I find the time to practice?** It's likely that you're spending a lot of time around your baby. You may not yet realize that so much of what you do with your baby includes a window of opportunity to learn and practice signing with them. Since your baby needs to be fed, changed, and bathed, you can incorporate practicing signing with your baby during your set routines. When you're about to feed, practice signing "Bottle" (page 72). When you're about to change their diaper, sign "Diaper" (page 114). When you're done bathing them, sign "Towel" (page 112). And repeat!

- **I'm trying to use sign language, but isn't my baby still too young to sign back?** Remind yourself of your goal: You want to communicate in sign language with your baby. With consistency of exposure, your baby will develop the ability to use sign language, just like they will eventually learn how to crawl or walk. Think about how rewarding it will be when your baby eventually signs back to you because you were consistent and kept at it.

- **How do I get my baby's attention?** Get on their level. If they're on their tummy, get on your tummy, too. If they are sitting, sit with them. If they're at the table, pull your chair near them. You can tap them or call their name to try to get them to look at you. Also, minimize potential distractions in the area. If there are toys around, put them away before you sign.

- **How do I get my baby to recognize a sign?** Whenever you sign with your baby, make sure you are signing something you see. You don't want to point at a tree and talk about what's for dinner. With the appropriate visual association to an object, person, or action while signing, you'll help your baby understand quicker.

- **How can I help my baby learn sign language other than by repetition?** Try guiding your baby's hands from underneath. Without forcing them to sign, guide their hands into a sign or the primary motion of a sign. By presenting gentle guidance from underneath your baby's hands, you give them the freedom to pull their hands away if desired.

When to Add On and When to Pause

Above all, learning and teaching ASL should be enjoyable and rewarding. If you or your baby get frustrated with signing at any point, take a
break so you don't get overwhelmed. If you and your baby are comfortable using certain signs, consider adding a few more new signs. There's
no timeline or deadline for using sign language with your baby. And no
one way works for everyone. When you and your baby aren't progressing
as quickly as you hoped, don't despair. Learning sign language is not a
linear process—it takes practice, consistency, and time.

You may realize that a certain sign you've been trying to use with
your baby isn't right for you. No worries! Discontinue that sign and try
working on another one. By trying another sign, you are seeing if it better
suits your communication needs. No matter how many or few signs you
and your baby learn to use, you'll be increasing communication and
understanding between the two of you.

What to Expect

You may wonder what to expect from your baby in using sign language.
Check out the "Child Development and Signing Milestones" sidebar
(page 16). This section shares some of what you can expect by age.
Generally, babies tend to start signing back between five and ten months
old. It may not always be crystal clear at first what your baby understands or what they are expressing in sign language. Your baby's first

Child Development and Signing Milestones

0-6 months

- Your baby's sight is still developing, so be sure to sign up close to them, where they can see you and your hands.

- Your baby is mostly working on skills like holding their head up, rolling over, and sitting up, so they probably won't be signing back yet.

- You may notice at some point that your baby is focusing on your hands, tracking your movements, and maybe even responding emotionally.

- Most babies do not start signing back during this age, so think of this as a time for you to practice signing and getting used to using a few starter signs consistently.

6-12 months

- Your baby may start to babble with their hands. These hand motions may not fully form accurate handshapes for particular signs. A common babbling movement you may see a baby do is batting their arms up and down repeatedly. If you've been signing to them, this signals that your baby is beginning to recognize their own ability to sign.

- While most signs may not be entirely accurate, a baby's first clear sign may begin to emerge. You can build upon that sign by reinforcing its use in practice.

- Try using animated facial expressions with your baby. This is a valuable part of communicating specific ideas.

- Your baby may begin to use their finger to point. If your baby points to something that you know the sign for, you can associate their pointing with the sign to help them acquire this sign.

12–18 months

- Your baby may be able to understand several separate one-word or two-word signs. Additionally, they may be able to express several one-word signs.

- Your baby may be able to pair a single sign with pointing. For instance, your baby may be able to point to you and sign "Mom" or point to a bottle and sign "Milk."

- To reiterate, continue signing the accurate sign, even if you see your baby signing handshapes or motions that are not yet accurate.

18–24 months

- Your child may begin to match an appropriate facial expression with a sign. For instance, they may frown and sign "Sad." If they make an appropriate facial expression for the sign they do, you can reinforce that by pointing to your child and asking, for example, if they are sad by signing "Sad" with a sad facial expression.

- Depending on when you started signing with your baby, they may now be able to sign many, if not most, of the signs in this book.

- Your child will likely produce a variety of facial expressions along with certain signs, like raising their eyebrows or squinting.

24–30 months

- Your child may be able to modify the signs they were signing inaccurately into signs that are accurate.

- You may notice your child begin to sign a variety of words during a conversation or while storytelling.

- If you and your child are communicating with all the words in this book, they may be ready for next steps. Take advantage of the resources section (page 150) for ways to learn more ASL.

signs might not look like the signs taught in this book. This doesn't mean that a baby is not able to sign. If a baby is moving their hands in a way they don't normally do, they may be signing to you in their own way!

For instance, a baby may not be able to accurately sign "I Love You" the way it's taught on page 64. The sign for "I Love You" includes sticking out your thumb, index finger, and pinkie with your dominant hand in front of your chest. Your baby may sign "I Love You" by sticking out their thumb and index finger but not their pinkie. If they haven't signed with that handshape before, you might be able to determine that they are trying to sign "I Love You." Sometimes you might not be sure. When you're not sure, wait and see if they do the same handshape at a later time.

Even if your baby is signing a word differently than is taught in this book, continue to sign the right way. With exposure to accurate signs, your baby will eventually modify and correct their own signs to become more similar to the signs you teach them.

Essential Tips for Signing Success

Every sign language journey plays out differently. To ensure that your experience with sign language is a positive one, incorporate sign language by weaving it into your day little by little. Learning sign language does not have to be intensive and serious. Take your time and enjoy the process!

- **Remember that every child's development and response are different.** As you use sign language with your baby, you'll learn what works best for both of you. Perhaps your baby does better learning signs in the morning than in the afternoon. Maybe your baby won't sign back to you until they are a year old. It's all okay. Every child acquires language in their own ways. Meet them where they are.

- **Use signs that are relevant to the context you are in.** Be sure to use signs that have to do with what's happening at the moment. If you are getting ready to go outside to play, for example, sign words and phrases that have to do with getting ready.

- **Try numerous ways to get your baby's attention.** Here are just a few: Wave your hand in their view to shift their focus to you. Tap their shoulder gently until they look at you. Hold the object of focus by your face so they look at you while you sign to them. If you're still not able to get their attention, it's okay to let them be and try again later.

- **Use your hands and facial expressions whenever you can.** You may not know the proper sign for something in the moment. In that case, resort to pointing or gesturing. Point to what you're talking about, gesture how to use an object, or express an emotion with a facial expression. You can look up the sign in this book later, or if it's not here, check out the resources (page 150) for guidance.

- **Don't be afraid to get moving while you're signing.** Sign language is highly interactive. Interaction will pique your baby's interest and motivation to engage with you. Teaching sign language does not involve any materials, just your hands. As you move from room to room or walk around a store, point at objects or people you're referring to. Show how you feel with facial expressions and body language.

- **Keep sign language fun and easy.** As you learn signs, insert a sign or two in each routine of the day, whether you're getting ready to go outside and play or changing your baby's diaper. Each chapter contains suggestions for incorporating sign language into your baby's daily activities.

- **Engage with every movement a baby makes with their hands.** Try to pay attention, even when your baby's movements seem to be spontaneous. It's essential to acknowledge when a baby is trying to communicate. With some guessing and observation of possible patterns over time, you may be able to recognize what your baby is signing to you. Show them that they have your full attention, and sign back to them in the context that seems relevant. This will encourage them to continue communicating with you. And then, one day soon, the light bulb will appear—you will understand them!

- **Work on consistency, habits, and routine.** When you sign consistently to your baby, even when there seems to be no progress made, signing will become a habit. Once this happens, you will be able to build sign language into your daily routines.

ASL for Babies FAQs

As you progress through this book, you may have questions. Read the following section for answers to some of the most common questions people pose regarding ASL for babies.

Q: How do I sign with my baby when I am holding them?

A: There are ways! Many signs only use one hand, though some signs use two. While it is important to maintain accuracy of signing, there are many cases (such as when holding a baby) when it's okay to adapt such signs. Ensure that you're positioned where your baby can see at least one hand. For any signs that are usually signed with two hands, use your free hand to sign what you would normally sign with your dominant hand.

Q: How can we incorporate signing as a bilingual family?

A: Since it is likely that you use more spoken words than signed words, try to do ASL-only with the words you know in ASL. For instance, if you know the sign for "Walk," sign it instead of verbally saying "walk." Your baby will have plenty of exposure to spoken language, since it is likely your primary mode of communication. When using just ASL for signs you know, you are allowing your baby to pick up ASL, too.

Q: Will using sign language delay speech development?

A: Children who solely use sign language or are bilingual with a spoken language and ASL are not more likely than other children to have delays in speech development. Regardless of what language your child acquires, they are developing an understanding of language. What they learn in ASL will reinforce and strengthen their foundation in speech and language development, rather than hinder it.

Q: My child has a learning disability. Do I need to adjust my approach around sign language?

A: No, you don't need to change your approach. In fact, using sign language with your child who has a learning disability may help further understanding, communication, and connection. Many people who have a disability find that using sign language is helpful in being able to communicate better.

Q: Should I stop signing once my baby starts talking?

A: If using ASL has been useful and rewarding for you and your baby, keep signing! Even when your baby starts talking, using sign language will continue to expose them to language enrichment. Using ASL with your baby has long-lasting benefits (see page 9).

Q: Do I need to make sure everyone in my baby's life is using sign language for it to stick?

A: Since your baby is primarily spending time with you, your baby will be able to learn and use ASL. Sure, it would be nice for anyone your baby interacts with to use sign language. However, that may not always be possible. To help bridge the gap, show other caregivers a few key signs to look for if you can. For example, it could prove useful for others to be familiar with the signs for "Hurt" and "Milk."

Q: My baby seems to be picking up one sign, but not another one. Why?

A: Babies learn and use language at various paces. Some babies use only one sign for a while before they show an interest in or pick up on another sign. As long as you continue to sign consistently with your baby, they will eventually pick up on other signs.

Q: I'm feeling discouraged. What if my baby never learns to sign back?

A: It's perfectly normal to feel discouraged at times. Like with most learned skills, learning a language takes time and practice. If you continue to use sign language daily and follow the suggestions and tips provided in this book, your baby will eventually sign back to you.

CHAPTER 2

Starter Signs

~~~~~~~~~~

This chapter covers 10 starter signs you may find most useful in communicating with your baby. The words "Milk," "Eat," and "All Done" are popular during a baby's mealtimes. This chapter also includes words such as "Thank You" and "Help." These words can help you and your baby communicate appreciation and personal needs.

Milk

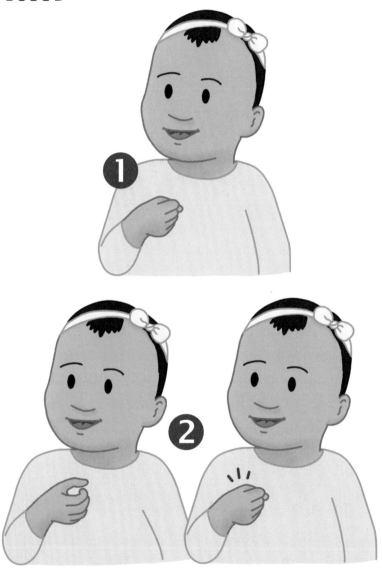

1 In front of your chest, form an upright closed fist and wrap your thumb outside and around your fingers. **2** Squeeze and release your fist slightly a few times.

How and When to Use This Sign

→ Prior to feeding your baby with milk, sign "Milk" with a questioning look on your face, asking them if they want milk.

→ Other words in this book that can be used with this sign include "Hot" (page 76) or "Cold" (page 78) if you provide milk via a bottle, to communicate the temperature of the milk.

Memory Hack
The sign for "Milk" is similar to milking a cow.

Helping Hand
You can assist your baby with this sign by placing their hand inside yours and gently squeezing the hand as you sign "Milk."

Eat

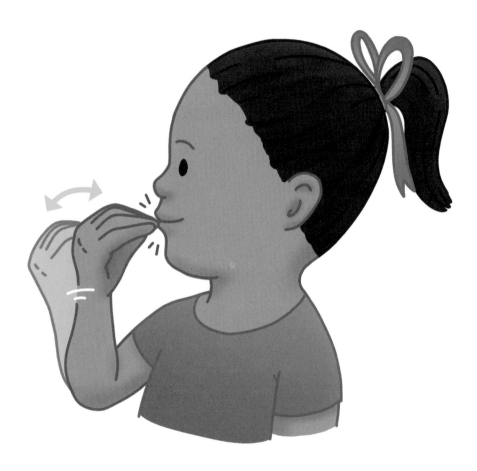

With your dominant hand, create the shape of an O. Flatten the O into a teardrop shape. With this formation, bring your hand toward your mouth, gently tapping your lips a couple of times with your fingertips.

How and When to Use This Sign

→ Point to your baby's food, then sign "Eat" with the same hand. You can repeat the sign with one hand as you feed your baby with the other hand.

→ The sign for "Eat" can also be used to sign "Food."

Memory Hack

The sign for "Eat" is similar to pinching several cashews with your fingers and placing them into your mouth.

Watch for This!

A baby may just point to any food, showing that they wish to eat, before they learn the sign for "Eat."

More

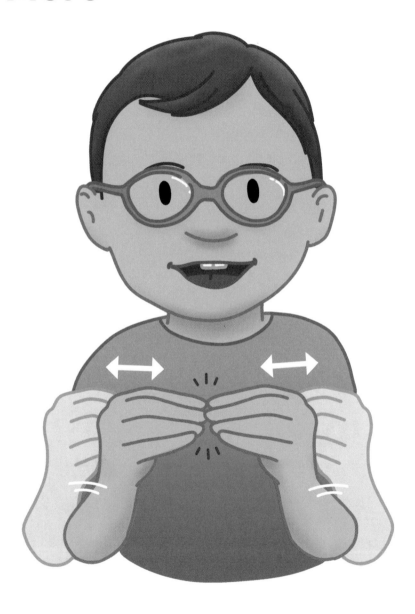

Learn to Sign with Your Baby

With each hand, create the shape of an O. Flatten each O into a teardrop shape. Gently peck the fingertips of both hands against each other a couple of times.

How and When to Use This Sign

→ Let's say you're feeding your baby puréed bananas. Each time you give your baby a spoonful, you can set the spoon down and sign "More?"

→ While there is a separate sign for "Again," you can also use the sign for "More" when something is to be done again.

Watch for This!
Look for the motion of two hands bumping into one another even if they are not formed into teardrop shapes. This is probably your baby signing "More."

Helping Hand
You can use the sign for "More" during playtime. If you're pushing your child on a swing, ask them if they would like to be pushed more while using the sign.

All Done

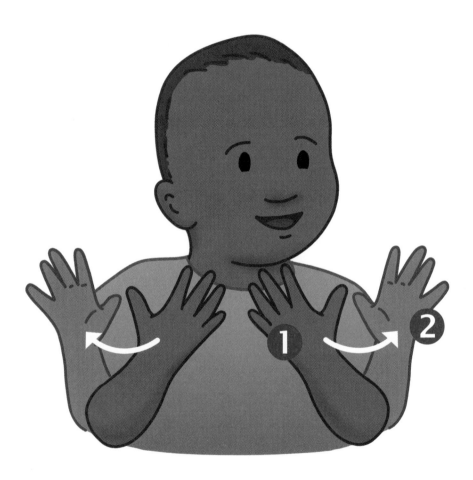

Learn to Sign with Your Baby

① In front of your chest, straighten out all 10 fingers with fingers spread out. Hold the fingertips facing up and palms facing your chest. **②** Rotate your wrists so your palms are now facing out. This motion is often repeated for emphasis.

How and When to Use This Sign

→ When it appears that your baby is done with an activity, sign "All Done." You can also use this word when all the milk in the bottle is gone.

Watch for This!
A baby may just raise their hands on either side of their body and shake them in various directions.

Helping Hand
Sign "All Done" with a proud grin followed by a high-five when your baby finishes stacking some blocks.

Please

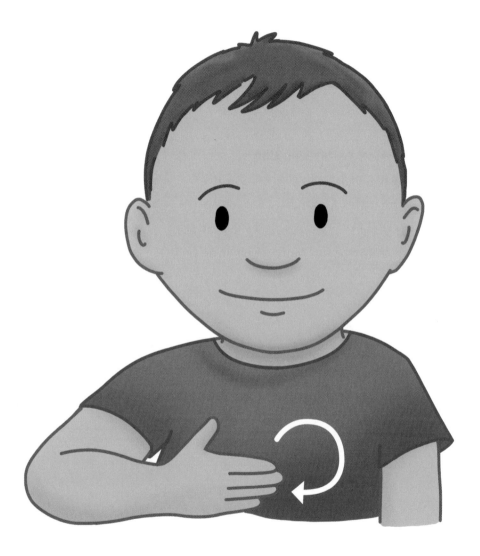

With your dominant hand, all fingers slightly spread out, press the inside of your palm at the center of your chest with the thumb facing up. While keeping your palm against your chest, create small circular motions against your chest.

How and When to Use This Sign

→ Use the sign for "Please" after you ask for something.

→ You can use the sign for "More" in combination with the sign "Please." For instance, your baby may sign "More please" when they wish to have more apples.

Memory Hack
Rub your heart warm with the flat of your palm.

Watch for This!
Use a flat hand when signing "Please" instead of a fist, because if you sign with a fist, that means "Sorry."

Thank You

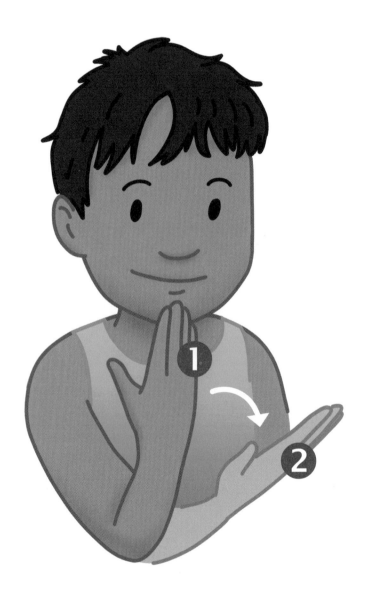

Learn to Sign with Your Baby

① With your dominant hand, straighten out all five fingers. Press your fingers together except for the thumb. Touch the front of your chin with the three middle fingers, palm facing you. **②** Keeping the wrist stationary, move your hand about a foot away from your chin.

How and When to Use This Sign

→ You can use this sign whenever you feel appreciation toward your baby. For example, if your baby offers you a toy or a bite of their food, sign "Thank You."

Watch for This!
Make sure you don't flick the bottom of your chin as you make the sign for "Thank You." That means something opposite to "thank you"!

Have Fun!
Guide your baby in signing "Thank You" to others in public who do nice things, such as holding the door open for you two.

Where

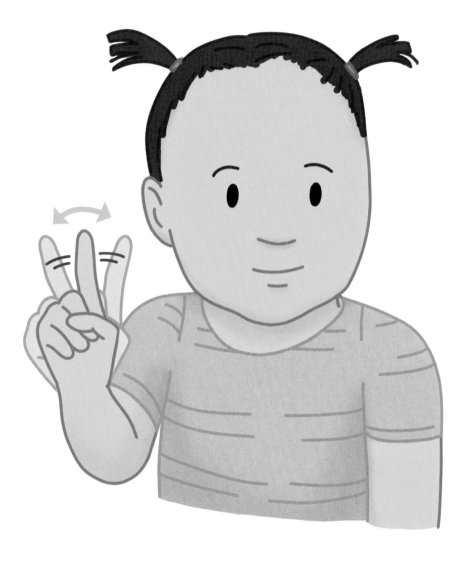

With your dominant hand, form a fist facing outward and straighten your index finger upward. Wag your wrist left and right slightly and quickly.

How and When to Use This Sign

→ Sign "Where" before you sign or say what you wish them to find or identify. You can also lower your eyebrows in an inquisitive way with this sign.

→ The sign for "Where" can be used in combination with signs found throughout this book. You can sign "Where" when you ask your baby where their shoes are, where the apples are, or where their toy duck is.

Memory Hack
Think about how people lick their index finger to feel what direction the wind is coming from.

Watch for This!
Your baby may just hold up one finger without wagging it back and forth when they are trying to sign "Where."

Help

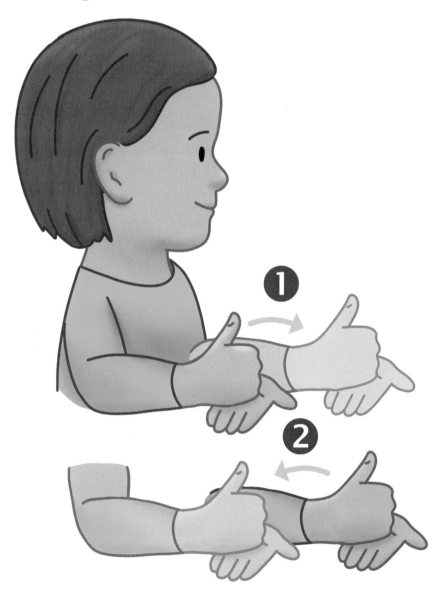

1 With your nondominant hand in front of your chest, hold out your palm flat, facing up. With your dominant hand, do a thumbs-up. Place the thumbs-up hand on top of the other hand. Extend your arms away from your body. This means you're offering help to your baby.

2 If you want help, bring the sign toward your chest.

How and When to Use This Sign

→ When you want your child to help clean up the toys, sign "Help" with movement toward your chest and point to the toys.

→ If they don't respond, you can pick up a few toys and put them away, then sign "Help" again.

Watch for This!
Your baby may sign "Help" with a closed fist rather than with a thumb sticking up.

Helping Hand
You can place a toy in your open palm while signing "Help" to show your child that this is what you want help with.

Another

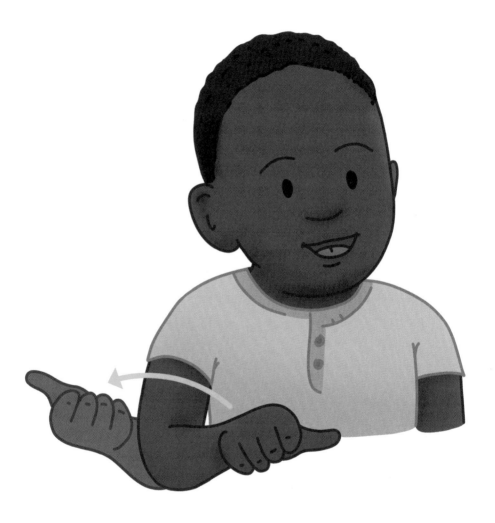

With your dominant hand, create a thumbs-up. Turn your wrist to the left (if left-handed) or to the right (if right-handed), so the thumbs-up turns sideways, pointing outward.

How and When to Use This Sign

→ If you have multiples of something such as books, after finishing a book, you can sign "Another."

Watch for This!
Make sure you sign "Another" with your thumb rotating outward rather than inward.

Have Fun!
If your baby takes another step forward as they learn how to walk, show facial excitement and sign "Another" to encourage another step.

My Turn/Your Turn

HANDSHAPE

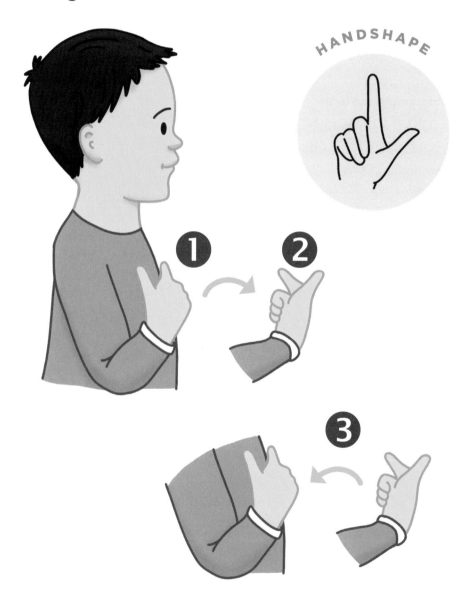

1 With your dominant hand, create an L shape. Place the L shape against the center of your chest, with your palm facing toward you, the index finger horizontal, and the thumb vertical. **2** Move the L away from your chest while simultaneously turning your wrist outward with a 90-degree turn. This means "Your Turn." **3** To sign "My Turn," maintain the handshape but do the opposite movement, starting in the finishing position and moving toward the chest.

How and When to Use This Sign

→ When you wish to take turns, sign "Your Turn" or "My Turn."

→ You might feed your baby a spoonful and then sign "My Turn" to communicate that it is your turn to eat a little bit of something, too.

Helping Hand
You can sign "Your Turn" with one hand while presenting a toy to your baby with the other hand at the same time.

Have Fun!
While at a store or playing outside, take turns pointing to things that are a particular color and sign "Your Turn" and "My Turn."

Family Pictures

SIGNS

- **Where** (p. 38)
- **Mom** (p. 50)
- **Dad** (p. 52)
- **Another** (p. 42)
- **My Turn/Your Turn** (p. 44)

This personal and sentimental activity is special to do with your baby because they will sense connection with those they know. All you need is a photo album that includes people your baby will recognize, such as parents, grandparents, siblings, and cousins.

1. Open your photo album to a picture of your immediate family, including your baby.

2. Sign "Where" and state a person's name, such as "Where is Mom?" Your baby then can point to who they think is Mom.

3. Next, you can ask, "Where is another picture of Mom?" while signing "Where" and "Another" and "Mom." When your baby points to another picture of Mom in the photo album, sign to them that it is "Your Turn" to turn the page.

4. Repeat steps 2 and 3 using other loved ones' names and taking turns turning the page.

Note: While you'll see "Mom" and "Dad" being used in this book as examples of a parent/caregiver name, please feel free to substitute whatever name your baby associates you with. See "Beyond 'Mom and Dad'" (page 53) for more on this.

A Visit to the Grocery Store

SIGNS

- **Help** (p. 40)
- **Apple** (p. 80)
- **Where** (p. 38)
- **Another** (p. 42)
- **More** (p. 30)
- **Please** (p. 34)
- **My Turn/Your Turn** (p. 44)
- **Thank You** (p. 36)
- **All Done** (p. 32)

This fun grocery store activity can be modified to your baby's mobility and level of communication. Here's an example of how it might go:

1. If your baby is not yet mobile, ask your baby, "Help me find the apples" while signing "Help" and "Apple." Your baby can point from where they are sitting or lying. It's okay if your baby doesn't know what apples look like. You can lead them to where the apples are, show them and sign "Apple," and place an apple in your cart.

2. Sign "Where" and "Apple" for "Where are the apples?"

3. Sign "Another" and "Apple" to say "We need another apple." (If your child is mobile and able to retrieve food, they could give you another apple.)

4. Sign "More" and "Please" and say, "We need more, please."

5. Sign "Your Turn" and "Another" and say, "It's your turn to pick out another fruit."

6. After your child points to or fetches another fruit, you can say, "Thank you. It's my turn to find some vegetables," while signing "Thank You" and "My Turn."

7. When you're done shopping, you can tell your child, "We're all done shopping!" while signing "All Done."

CHAPTER 3

People and Feelings

～～～～～～～～

Imagine how you would feel if your baby addressed you by name. Now imagine if they could do so in sign language! In this chapter, you'll learn about signs for parents and caregivers as well as for feelings such as happy and hurt. By teaching your baby ways to communicate how they feel, you'll gain a deeper understanding of their thoughts and emotions. During bath time, your baby may get some soap in their eye and sign "Hurt." To understand why they hurt, you may sign "Soap" (page 122) to see if they got soap in their eye. With their affirming nod, you'll have a baby who feels understood!

Mom

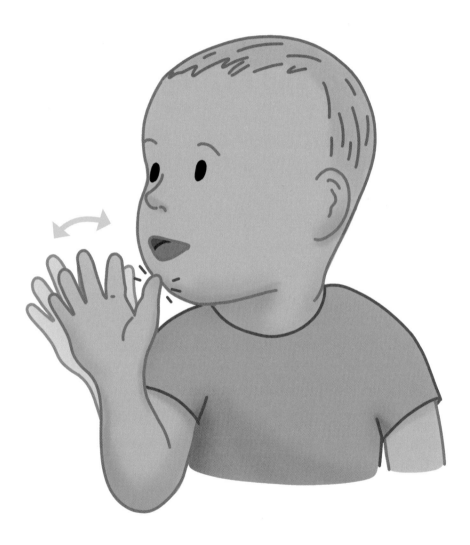

Learn to Sign with Your Baby

With your dominant hand, straighten and spread all five fingers. Tap the tip of your thumb a couple times against the middle of your chin.

How and When to Use This Sign

→ If you are Mom, when you wish to sign "Mom," point to yourself and then sign "Mom." By pointing first, you identify who you're talking about. If someone else is Mom, you can point to them and then sign "Mom."

→ You can combine many signs in this book with the sign for "Mom." For instance, you can sign "Mom" and then "Tired" (page 100) to indicate to your baby that you are tired.

Helping Hand

If you repeat the sign for "Mom" in different contexts, ·your baby will catch on more quickly. This applies to all signs you continuously repeat.

Watch for This!

Your baby may tap their palm or any other part of their hand against their chin rather than tapping the tip of their thumb on their chin.

Dad

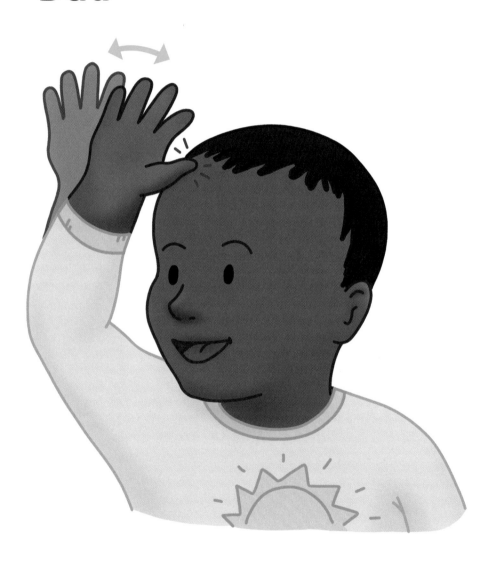

With your dominant hand, straighten and spread all five fingers. Tap the tip of your thumb a couple of times against the middle of your forehead.

How and When to Use This Sign

→ If you are Dad, point to yourself and then sign "Dad." If someone else is Dad, you can point to them and then sign "Dad."

→ If you want to help your baby sign "Dad," you can point to yourself and then guide their hand to their forehead. It's okay if they don't spread their fingers or use their thumb.

Beyond "Mom and Dad"

Not all caregivers or parents are called "Mom" or "Dad." You may be a caregiver who isn't a parent or a parent who doesn't identify within the binary of a "mom" or "dad." In such cases, a "sign name" can be used. For instance, if a caregiver's name starts with an L, a sign name might include signing "L" and shaking it back and forth a couple of times. It's important to remember that this is not an official sign. It's a "home sign," which means it's understood by those who use it and know who they're using it for.

Watch for This!
Your baby may touch the top of their head to sign "Dad."

Helping Hand
When you sign "Dad," turn your body and head sideways to show the sign more clearly to your baby. This will help them see the handshape and where you place it.

Baby

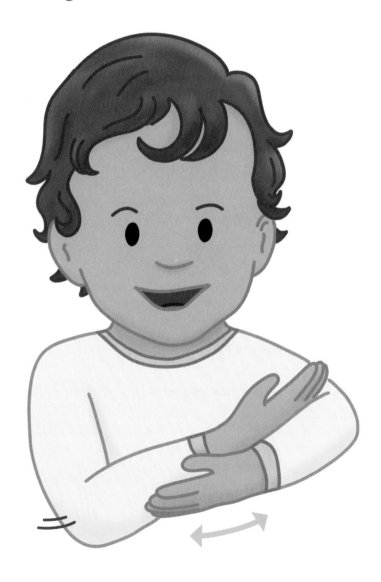

Bend both arms until they are at 90-degree angles. Put one arm on top of the other, with the top arm's fingers resting inside the crook of your other arm's elbow. Relax your shoulders and rock your arms back and forth, with your arms floating across your chest.

How and When to Use This Sign

→ Point to your baby and sign "Baby." If there is another baby around, you can also point to that baby and sign "Baby."

→ You can sign "Baby" with signs like "Happy" or "Sad." To do this, sign "Baby" with a questioning look on your face, and ask them "Happy?" or "Sad?" with the appropriate sign.

Memory Hack
The sign for a baby is like rocking a baby.

Have Fun!
When playing house, place a doll or stuffed animal inside both your and your baby's arms as though you're both rocking a baby.

Happy

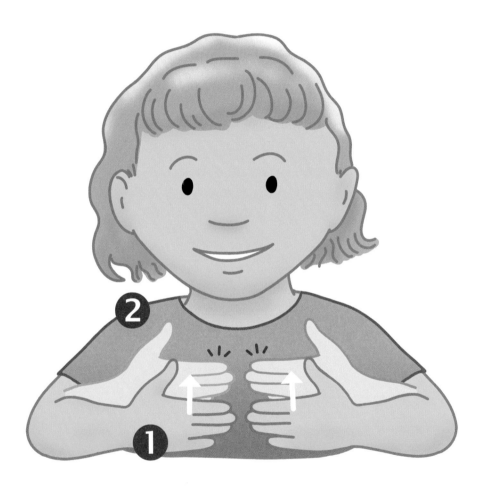

❶ With one hand, extend all five fingers. Press your fingers together except for the thumb, keeping your hand and fingers relaxed. **❷** With thumb up and palm facing your chest, brush the inside of your hand upward against your chest a couple of times. You may see variations to this sign, such as two hands doing the same motion.

How and When to Use This Sign

→ Sign "Happy" when you wish to tell your baby you feel happy, like after the baby gives you a hug and it makes you happy.

→ Since you are expressing an emotion in sign, also show that emotion with your body language and facial expressions. In this case, bring on your best smile!

Watch for This!
Make sure you sign "Happy" by brushing upward against your chest instead of downward.

Helping Hand
Usually we use words like "happy" for human emotion, but you can also sign "Happy" to describe a pet's emotion, such as when they get a treat.

Hurt

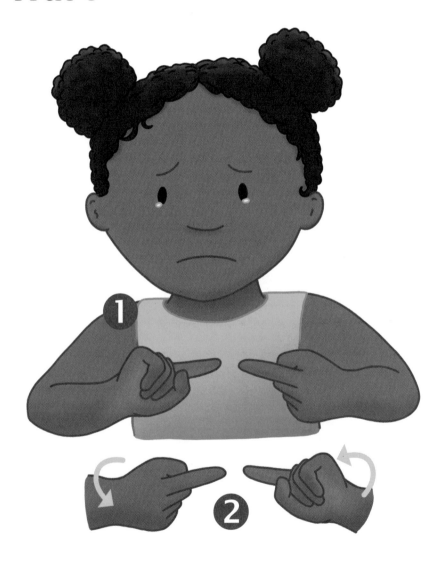

1 Create fists with both hands and stick out both index fingers. Point the tips of your index fingers at each other horizontally about an inch apart. **2** Twist your wrists slightly, with the dominant hand twisting in one direction and the nondominant hand twisting in the opposite direction.

How and When to Use This Sign

→ Sign "Hurt" where you are hurting. For instance, if you have a stomachache, sign "Hurt" in front of your stomach. If you scraped your knee, sign "Hurt" by the scrape.

→ If your baby is hurting, sign "Hurt" on yourself; for example, sign by your own knee when asking your baby if they bumped their knee. When you ask your baby if they are hurting but you're not sure where, sign "Hurt" in front of your chest.

Watch for This!
Your baby may sign "Hurt" with both index fingers touching one another, with or without the twisting motion.

Helping Hand
Make a hurt face as you do this sign.

Hug

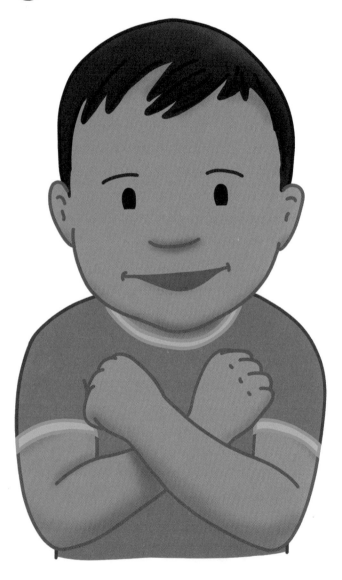

Form relaxed fists with both hands. Cross your arms over your chest. The fisted handshapes should be on either side of your chest, one on each side of the chest.

How and When to Use This Sign

→ When you wish to give or ask for a hug, sign "Hug."

→ To emphasize a passionate hug, you can cross your fists tightly across your chest and wiggle your body side to side. This communicates with body language that you wish to give a tight, wiggly hug.

Memory Hack
The sign for "Hug" is just like giving yourself a hug.

Helping Hand
Place your baby on your lap with them facing away from you. You can take their fists into your hands and cross their arms across their chest as you give them a hug from behind!

Sad

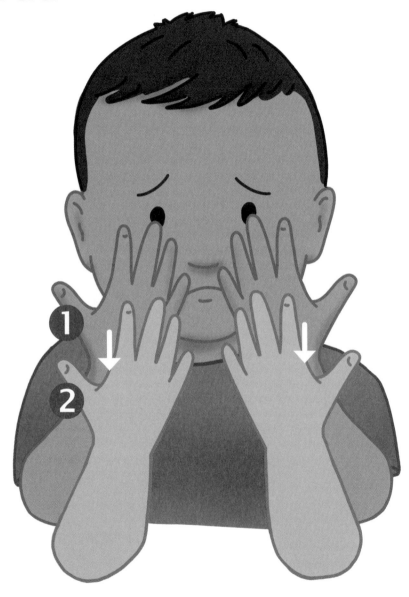

Learn to Sign with Your Baby

1 With both hands, straighten out all five fingers with fingers spread out, with your palms facing your face and fingertips up.

2 Bring down both hands until your hands are just above your chest.

How and When to Use This Sign

→ Sign "Sad" when you want to tell your baby you are feeling sad.

→ As you sign "Sad," show the emotion with body language (shoulders drooping inward) and facial expressions (frowning and furrowing your eyebrows).

Memory Hack
The sign for "Sad" is similar to tears rolling down your cheeks.

Watch for This!
Your baby may only use one hand to sign "Sad." (This is a possibility for all signs that are signed with two hands.)

I Love You

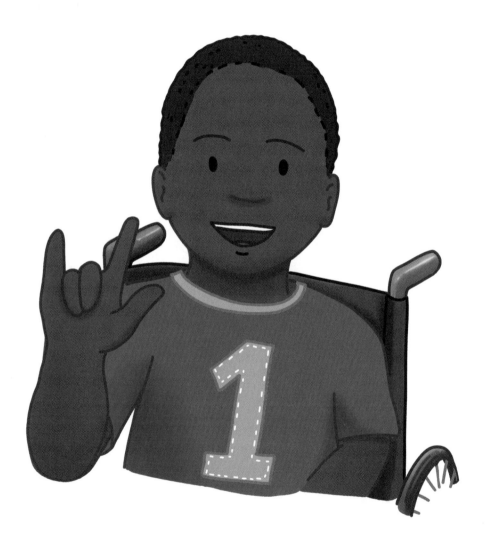

Learn to Sign with Your Baby

With your dominant hand, bend your middle and ring finger while keeping the remaining fingers straight. With this shape, place your hand comfortably in front of your dominant shoulder, palm facing out. You may see another way to sign this phrase, but this way condenses all three words into one sign.

How and When to Use This Sign

→ Sign "I Love You" when you wish to tell your baby you love them.

→ To emphasize your love, you can wiggle the handshape for "I Love You" a few times.

Memory Hack
The sign for "I Love You" includes the letters *I, L,* and *Y*!

Watch for This!
Since the sign for "I Love You" is a bit more complicated than other signs, your baby may sign just a Y shape or an L shape instead of making the proper hand-shape for "I Love You." You can bet they still love you, though!

I Spy Sign!

SIGNS

- **Mom** (p. 50)
- **Dad** (p. 52)
- **Happy** (p. 56)
- **Sad** (p. 62)
- **Hurt** (p. 58)
- **I Love You** (p. 64)
- **Where** (p. 38)

"I Spy!" is a game where you look for specific objects among many other objects. This version of the game is called "I Spy Sign!" This activity is wonderful because children like it when they see something similar done by other children. You'll need a laptop or tablet with internet access.

1. Go to giphy.com/aslnook. Scroll down to the ASL Nook GIFs.

2. Before showing your baby, look through the list of ASL Nook GIFs. You'll see parents and their children signing different words for a GIF. Look through the GIFs and find the following words taught in this chapter: "Mom," "Dad," "Happy," "Sad," "Hurt," and "I Love You."

3. Share the screen with your child. If you want them to find the GIF that signs "Happy," scroll down to where you see that GIF without pointing it out. You can ask them "Where" is the sign for "Happy"? Feel free to help them as needed.

4. Repeat for the remaining signs in the list above.

Am I Happy or Sad?

SIGNS

- **Sad** (p. 62)
- **Happy** (p. 56)
- **Hug** (p. 60)

Being able to express feelings is an important skill for life! This activity will help you teach your baby how to identify and communicate how they feel. There are no materials needed for this activity. All you need to know is how to make stellar facial expressions!

1. Position your baby in a safe space where they can look at you.

2. Make a face that shows that you're sad (or happy) and ask your baby what they think you're feeling. You can ask them "Am I sad?" (while signing "Sad") or "Am I happy?" (while signing "Happy"). It's okay if they don't sign "Sad" or "Happy" in response. Observe their body language and facial expressions. They may be responding in other ways for now.

3. To help them practice, you can answer for them by signing "Sad."

4. After you or your baby responds, you can ask for a hug by signing "Hug." This helps a baby learn the importance of caring for someone in response to their feelings. (But if they don't want to hug, that's okay, too!)

CHAPTER 4

Mealtimes

〜〜〜〜〜

We all have different mealtime preferences: Some like savory, some sweet, some cold, some hot. So does your baby. So how do you create a pleasant mealtime for them? How can you communicate needs during mealtime? That's right, by signing with your baby! In this chapter, you'll teach your baby how to communicate their preferences. Other useful signs for mealtimes include "Eat" (page 28), "More" (page 30), and "All Done" (page 32).

Drink

HANDSHAPE

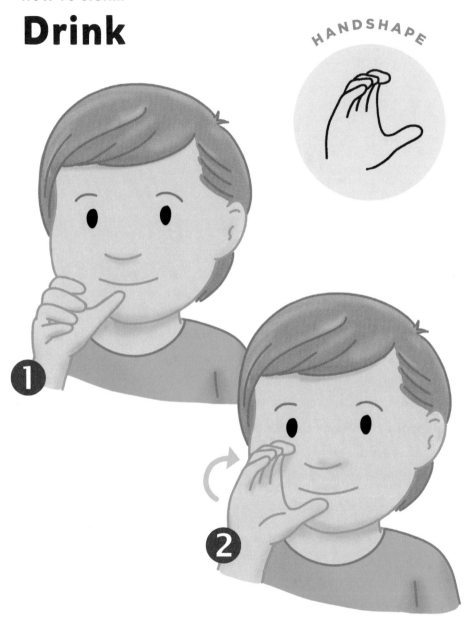

① With your dominant hand, create a C shape. **②** Tilt the C shape toward your mouth, with the thumb in front of your bottom lip and the other curved fingers hovering above your nose.

How and When to Use This Sign

→ Use the sign for "Drink" as you lift your cup to your lips.

→ You can sign "Another" with "Drink" to show your baby how to ask for another drink.

The sign for "Drink" mimics the action of bringing a glass to your lips.

Helping Hand
To help your baby connect the sign to their drink, hold their sippy cup or bottle next to your mouth with your non-dominant hand while signing "Drink" with your dominant hand.

Bottle

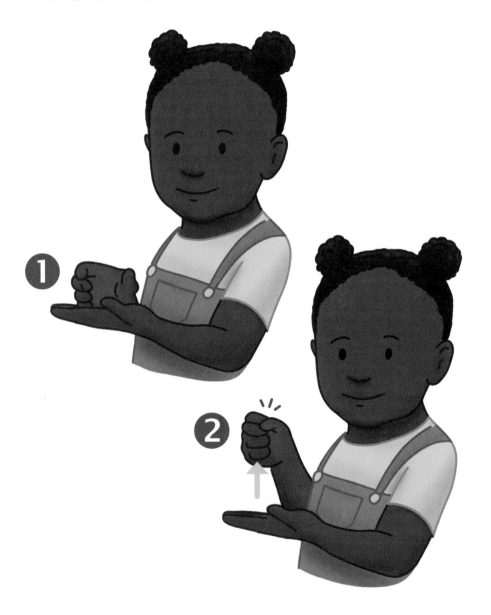

① Place your nondominant hand in front of your chest, hand flat and palm facing up, all fingers touching except for your thumb. With your dominant hand, place a C shape on its side and place it on top of the nondominant hand's palm, with the pinkie of the C resting lightly on the palm. **②** Lift the C shape away from the palm by a few inches, and contract the C shape into a fist.

How and When to Use This Sign

→ When you're about to feed your baby by bottle, point to the bottle and sign "Bottle."

→ Since you'll need both hands to sign "Bottle," do the sign before picking up your baby to feed them.

Watch for This!
Your baby may make an O instead of a C with their hand and place it on top of their other hand.

Helping Hand
You can place your baby's bottle on your nondominant palm and form a C shape around your baby's bottle with your other hand.

Spoon

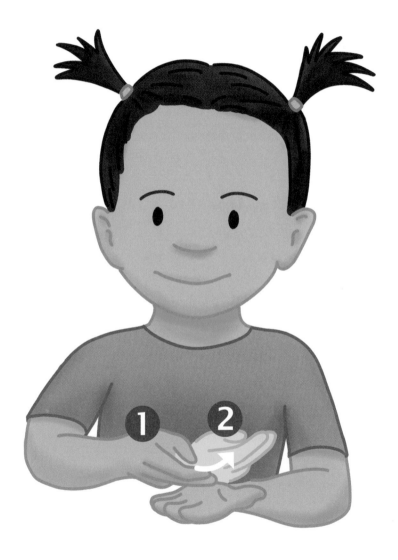

1 With your nondominant hand, make a relaxed cupped palm in front of your chest, facing up. With your dominant hand, create a fist with the palm up. Stick out your middle and index fingers in a relaxed, curved shape, fingers touching. **2** Brush these fingers in the middle of the nondominant hand's palm and make a scooping motion with the dominant hand about two inches up toward your mouth, and repeat once.

How and When to Use This Sign

→ Sign "Spoon" right before fetching one or feeding your baby with a spoon.

→ To help your baby associate the sign with the utensil, hold the spoon in your dominant hand and make the scooping motion for the sign with your other hand.

Memory Hack
The scooping motion you make for "Spoon" is similar to the way you would scoop up some soup, cereal, or yogurt.

Helping Hand
While your baby holds their spoon or feeds themself with a spoon, sign "Spoon."

Hot

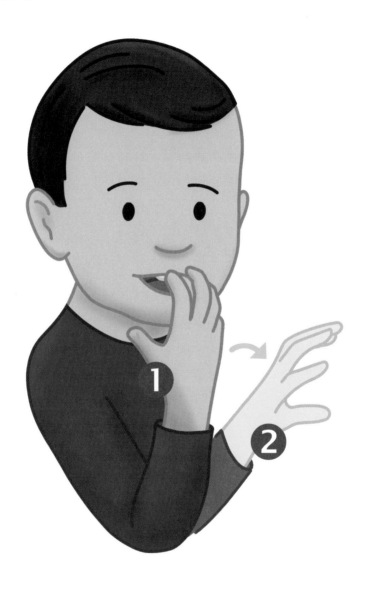

1 With your dominant hand, bend all fingers slightly inward as though you're gripping a doorknob with all fingers. Hold the bent fingers in front of your mouth, fingertips facing your mouth. **2** Turn your wrist until the handshape moves away from your mouth and faces outward in the opposite direction.

How and When to Use This Sign

→ Sign "Hot" when you touch, eat, or drink something hot.

→ Use body language and facial expressions to communicate that something is hot. To let your baby know their food is hot, you can touch the bowl and pull your arm back swiftly while making a sizzling sound with your clenched teeth as you sign "Hot."

Watch for This!
Your baby may not twist their wrist. They may just make the handshape and keep it at their mouth.

Helping Hand
Many caregivers use the sign for "Hot" for food, but you can also use it when you test the water for a bath.

Cold

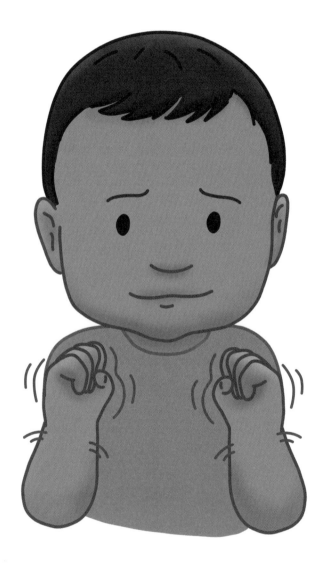

In front of your chest, hold both hands in tight fists, thumbs wrapping each fist and facing each other. Shiver the fists and forearms back and forth slightly but swiftly, without touching the fists together. You don't need to move your elbows or shoulders while doing this shivering motion.

How and When to Use This Sign

→ Sign "Cold" if you touched, ate, or drank something cold.

→ Use your body language and facial expressions to communicate when something is cold. To let your baby know their milk is cold, you can touch the bottle, pull back, and shiver with your body while chattering your teeth.

Memory Hack
The sign for "Cold" is much like the feeling of shivering.

Helping Hand
To practice these signs, you can ask your baby if it's hot or cold outside, or if the food you buy at the grocery store is hot or cold.

Apple

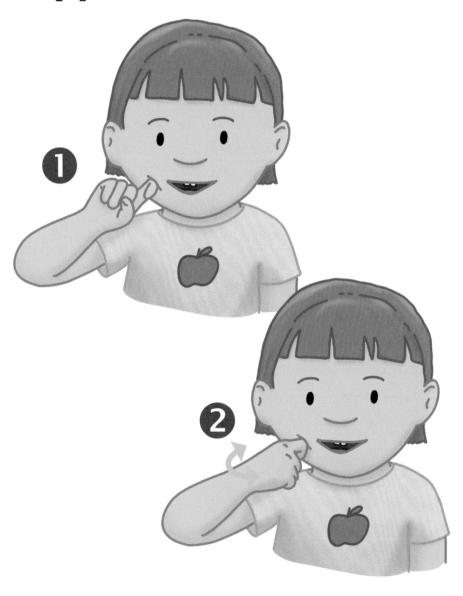

Learn to Sign with Your Baby

1 With your dominant hand, form a relaxed fist and straighten out your index finger. Bend your index finger, creating a relaxed hook. Place the outside knuckle of your bent index finger on the middle of your cheek. **2** Twist your wrist forward slightly, and repeat the motion once more.

How and When to Use This Sign

→ When you show your baby you're going to give them some apples, sign "Apple."

→ After they've had a bite, you can ask them if they want more, using the signs for "More" (page 30) and "Apple."

Helping Hand
If you're making homemade apple purée, sign "Apple" a few times as you cut up the apple, cook it, and purée it.

Have Fun!
Go to your nearest apple orchard and pick your own apples. Sign a lot of "Apple" while you enjoy your family outing!

Banana

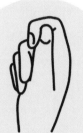

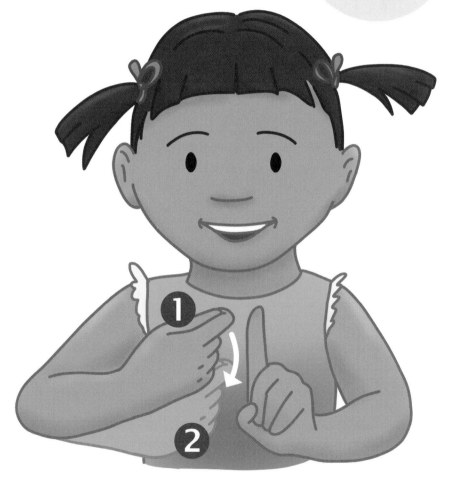

Learn to Sign with Your Baby

1 With your nondominant hand, form a fist and straighten your index finger. Hold this handshape out in front of your chest, fingertip pointing up. With your dominant hand, bend your index finger halfway down. Place the tip of your dominant thumb against the bent index fingertip. **2** Brush your bent index finger against the index finger on your nondominant hand, from top to bottom. Repeat, brushing another side of your index finger.

How and When to Use This Sign

→ When you present your baby with some bananas to eat, sign "Banana."

→ Ask your baby if they would like more, using the signs for "More" (page 30) and "Banana."

Memory Hack
The sign for "Banana" is much like the action of peeling a banana.

Watch for This!
Make sure you use your index finger on your nondominant hand when you sign "Banana." Some may accidentally use a different finger.

Hungry

HANDSHAPE

1 With your dominant hand, create a C shape. Place the C shape at the top of your chest, with the fingertips and tip of your thumb touching your chest. **2** Slide the handshape downward in the middle of your chest until you reach halfway down your torso.

How and When to Use This Sign

→ When you ask your baby if they are hungry, point to them with a questioning facial expression and sign "Hungry?"

→ If you want to emphasize hunger, give a big sigh and let your body bounce downward a bit as you sign "Hungry."

Memory Hack

The sign and motion for "Hungry" is similar to the action of food going down to your stomach.

Have Fun!

If you have a pet, sign "Hungry" to your baby and point at your pet right before feeding them. You can also do this while your pet is gobbling up their food—you may get your baby giggling!

Wash

HANDSHAPE

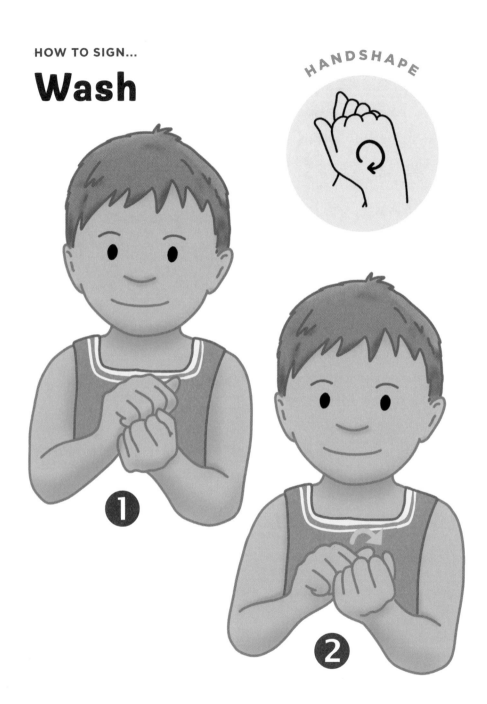

Learn to Sign with Your Baby

1 With both hands, create fists, thumbs touching the sides of your fists by the index fingers. Turn your nondominant fist so the fingers are facing up. Do the opposite with your dominant hand. Rest the dominant fist on the nondominant fist with the fingers facing each other. **2** Turn your dominant top hand in small circular motions while still touching the bottom hand.

How and When to Use This Sign

→ Before wiping your baby's face with a washcloth, sign "Wash" and show them the washcloth.

→ Let your baby hold the washcloth and try washing their face while you sign "Wash" encouragingly.

Memory Hack
The sign for "Wash" is much like the action of washing dishes.

Helping Hand
Many parents use "Wash" at the end of mealtimes or bath time, but you can also use it when you're wiping down their high chair.

Stop

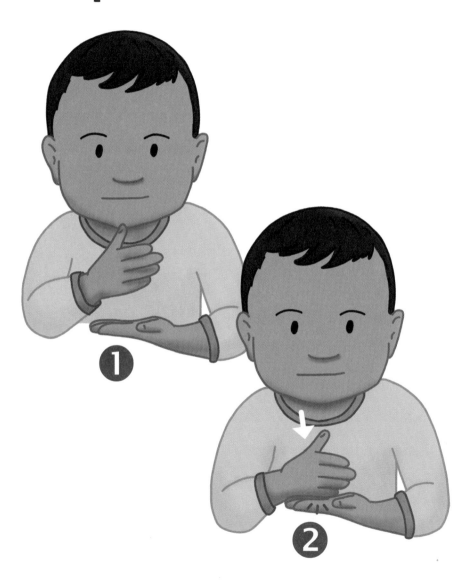

Learn to Sign with Your Baby

1 Hold your nondominant hand flat in front of your chest, palm up and fingers straight and touching except the thumb. Create the same handshape for your dominant hand, palm facing sideways. **2** Lower your dominant hand perpendicularly onto the middle of your nondominant hand, with the side of the pinkie touching your nondominant hand.

How and When to Use This Sign

→ If your baby is doing something you don't want them to do, sign "Stop." Depending on how serious you are about them stopping, you can sign "Stop" more swiftly.

→ You can use the sign "Please" (page 34) before signing "Stop" to provide a more pleasant interaction while still being firm about your wishes.

Watch for This!
Your baby may do this sign with just one hand by swinging down their hand similar to the motion of the dominant hand.

Have Fun!
You can sign "Stop" whenever you and your baby encounter a stop sign on a walk. No stop signs? No problem—just stop spontaneously on your walk and sign "Stop."

Bring a Friend!

SIGNS

- **Apple** (p. 80)
- **Spoon** (p. 74)
- **Wash** (p. 86)
- **Any or all of the signs in chapter 4**

How fun would it be for your baby to bring their favorite plushie to mealtime? The purpose of this activity is to role-play in sign language with something that is important and personal to your baby—in this case, their special plush friend. All you need is your baby's plushie, some applesauce, and two bowls, spoons, and/or bottles or sippy cups—whatever dishes you use for your baby during mealtime—along with a washcloth.

1. Set your baby's plushie nearby, where they can see it, and place one set of dishes in front of the plushie.

2. First, pretend-feed the plushie. Use any of the signs in chapter 4 to "communicate" with your baby's plushie. Let your baby observe the signs you use and why you're using them. For example, ask the plushie if they want applesauce by signing "Apple." Next, sign "Spoon" as you scoop the applesauce and pretend-feed the plushie.

3. Next, turn to your baby and ask if they want applesauce by signing "Apple." You can then repeat what you did with your baby's plushie, signing "Spoon" and feeding them. Take turns "feeding" plushie and baby.

4. End the meal by signing "Wash" and wiping your baby and plushie with a warm washcloth.

Food Explorer

SIGNS

- **Banana** (p. 82)
- **Cold** (p. 78)
- **Another** (p. 42)
- **More** (p. 30)

Did you know that sensory activities help stimulate a baby's reflexes, especially in their first year? With this activity, you'll combine sensory play with sign language! This activity doesn't need to be done around mealtime but can bolster communication surrounding meal-related signs. All you need are bananas, an ice cube tray, and a bowl.

1. Cut one or two bananas into thick slices (for ease of grabbing).
2. Put half of the banana slices in the freezer and let them get cold.
3. After the bananas from the freezer turn cold, put all the banana slices, including the room-temperature slices, into a shallow bowl.
4. Sit your baby in their high chair or at the table. Sit down with them. Place the bowl of bananas in front of you while placing the empty ice cube tray in front of your baby.
5. Ask your baby if they would like a banana while signing "Banana." Pick up a banana slice and give it to them. Ask them if it is cold while signing "Cold." If it is not cold, shake your head back and forth side to side. Guide them to put the banana in one of the empty wells of the ice cube tray.
6. Ask your baby if they would like another banana using the signs for "Another" or "More." Ask them again if the banana is cold by signing "Cold." Guide them to put the banana in another ice cube well. Continue as long as desired.

CHAPTER 5

Sleeping and Rising

~~~~~~~~~~~~~~~~

Bedtime and morning routines can be challenging. But they don't have to be! By signing with your baby, you may have an easier time getting into a comfortable routine. Imagine your baby becoming accustomed to you signing "Toothbrush" followed by "Bed"—this way they know what's coming. Once their little front teeth are clean and they are brought to bed, you then sign "Blanket" as you tuck them into their cozy space. Before turning off the lights, you smile and sign a sweet "Goodnight." With clear communication, your baby will know what's happening. They can go to sleep feeling secure, knowing they have been put to bed like this before.

Good Morning

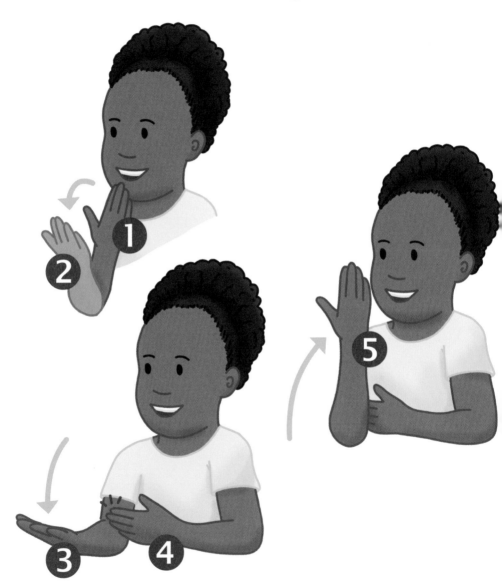

This two-part phrase has two separate signs done consecutively. **1** To sign "Good," create a flat handshape with your dominant hand, palm up, fingers touching, and thumb sticking out. Place the inside of your fingertips on the front of your chin. **2** Bring this handshape away from your chin slightly. **3** To sign "Morning," maintain the handshape for "Good" and extend your dominant elbow to a 90-degree angle. **4** While doing this, create the same handshape with your nondominant hand. Place this handshape in the crook of your dominant hand's elbow. **5** Bring the dominant handshape up toward your face, stopping once the handshape in your elbow is slightly pinched. Sign "Good" and "Morning" consecutively, without a pause in between.

How and When to Use This Sign

→ When you wake your baby (or they wake you!) in the morning, sign "Good Morning."

→ To start the day off right, you can sign "Good Morning" in a chipper manner, emphasizing the sign for "Good Morning."

Watch for This!

Your baby may do this sign with one hand by bringing up their hand similar to the motion of the dominant hand.

Helping Hand

If there are others in your home, you can sign "Good Morning" to them with your baby as you see them.

Goodnight

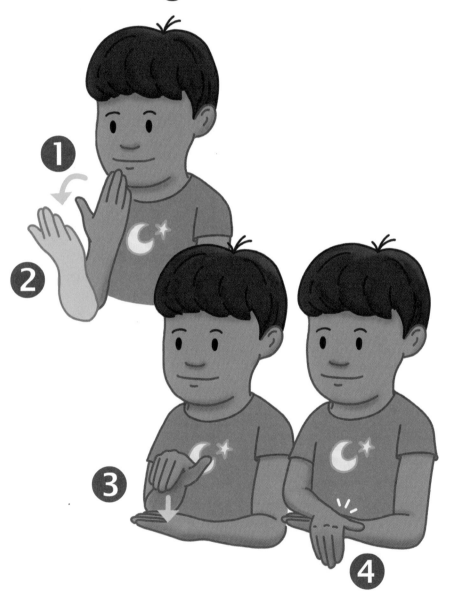

This phrase has two separate signs done consecutively. **1** To sign "Good," create a flat handshape with your dominant hand, palm up, fingers touching and thumb sticking out. Gently place the inside of your fingertips on the front of your chin. **2** Bring this handshape away from your chin slightly. **3** For "Night," create a bowl-like shape with your dominant hand. Your dominant hand's thumb should be sticking out. With your nondominant hand, create a flat handshape with the thumb relaxed. Hold both hands in front of your chest, palms down, and the dominant hand hovering over the nondominant hand. **4** Bring down the inside of your dominant hand's wrist until it touches the top of your nondominant hand's wrist. Sign "Good" and "Night" consecutively, without a pause in between.

How and When to Use This Sign

→ When you put your baby to bed and before you turn off the lights, sign "Goodnight."

→ To suggest that it's time to be quiet and rest, sign "Goodnight" in a soft, gentle manner.

Helping Hand

You can sign "Goodnight" to your baby's plushie and then sign "Goodnight" to your baby as you tuck them in.

Have Fun!

Call a loved one on a video call and sign "Goodnight" to them with your baby. Encourage the loved one to sign back.

Bed

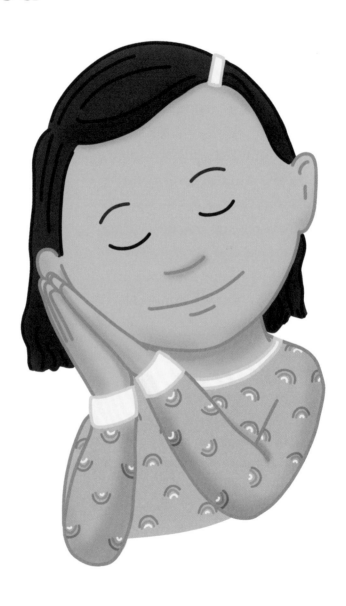

Learn to Sign with Your Baby

With both hands, straighten out your fingers so they are touching and your thumbs are pressing the side of the hands. Touch the palms of both hands together, with all fingers parallel to one another. Bring this handshape to your cheek on the dominant side, with the surface of the closest hand to the face touching the cheek and head.

How and When to Use This Sign

→ Sign "Bed" to signal when it's time for bed.

→ You can point to your baby's crib and sign "Bed." You also can sign "Bed" for any place you plan to sleep (such as a couch) or when it is naptime.

Memory Hack
The sign for "Bed" is like the action of resting your head on a surface.

Watch for This!
Your baby may sign "Bed" with one hand to the side of their face. This is actually another way to sign "Bed" more casually. You can use this sign if that works best for you and your baby.

Tired

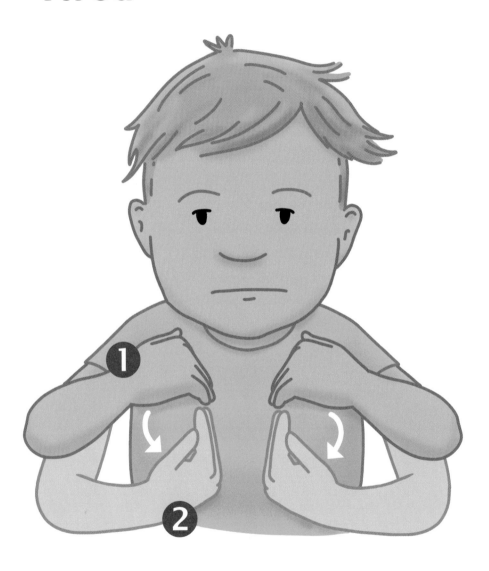

Learn to Sign with Your Baby

1 With both hands, create a C shape. Relax the C shapes into bowl shapes and place the fingertips on top of your chest. **2** Twist your wrists downward until the pinkie side is pressing against the chest and the thumb side is facing out.

How and When to Use This Sign

→ When you feel tired, point to the middle of your chest and sign "Tired." Use body language to show that you are tired.

→ You can sign "Bed" after "Tired" to communicate that you're going to nap or sleep.

Watch for This!
Your baby may put their two hands on top of their chest rather than doing the full motion for "Tired."

Helping Hand
The signs for feeling words like "tired" are most effective when accompanied by body language— in this case, a tired face and sagging shoulders.

Blanket

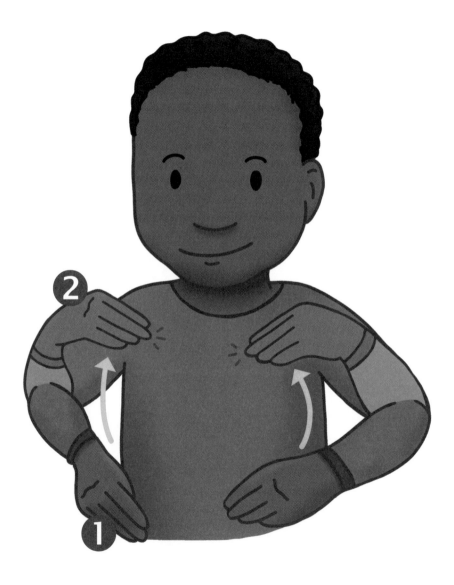

1 With both hands, stick out all your fingers, touching, except for the thumb. Stick out your thumbs until they're hovering beneath your other fingers. Hover these handshapes in front of your stomach, palms facing your body.

2 Bring both handshapes up to your chest, eventually touching your thumbs to the fingers above them.

How and When to Use This Sign

→ Before tucking in your baby or putting a blanket over them, sign "Blanket."

→ You can use the signs for "Hot" (page 76) and "Cold" (page 78) with this sign if you want to ask your baby if they are hot or cold.

Memory Hack
The sign for "Blanket" is like the action of pulling up a blanket over your chest.

Helping Hand
You can use this sign with an inquisitive look when you tuck your baby in the stroller or sit down to read a book together, as if to ask, "Would you like a blanket?"

Toothbrush

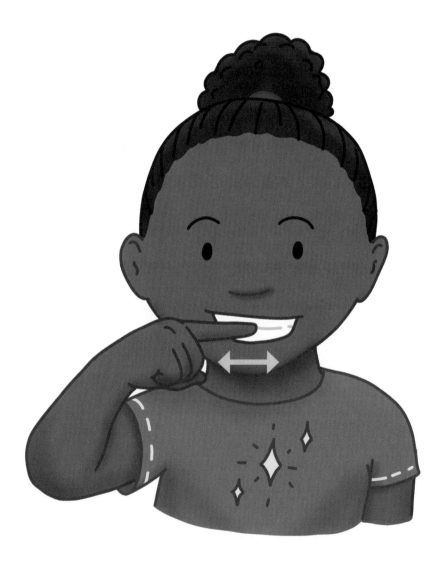

Learn to Sign with Your Baby

With your dominant hand, create a fist and stick out your index finger. As you do, clench your teeth together and show them. Bring your index finger in front of and parallel to your lips and exposed teeth. Slide your index finger slightly back and forth across the front of your mouth a few times.

How and When to Use This Sign

→ When it's time to brush your baby's new pearly whites, sign "Toothbrush."

→ Sign "Toothbrush" with your dominant hand as you pick up their toothbrush with your nondominant hand.

Memory Hack
The sign for "Toothbrush" is much like the action of brushing your teeth.

Helping Hand
To encourage good dental habits from an early age, brush baby's teeth after each bottle or meal—and don't forget to sign "Toothbrush"!

Ready

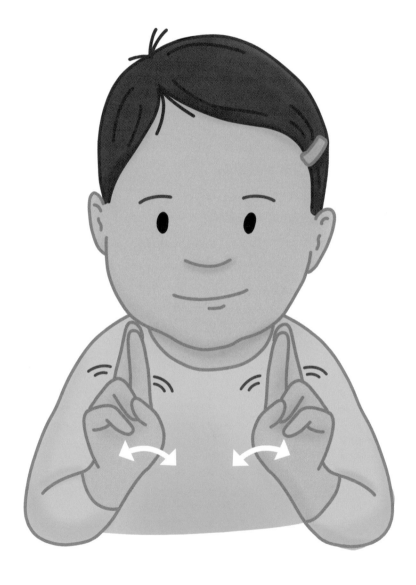

Learn to Sign with Your Baby

With both hands, create fists and stick out your index and middle fingers. Twist your middle fingers over top of your index fingers. This creates the letter *R*. Place these handshapes in front of your chest without touching one another. Gently wiggle both handshapes back and forth in front of you.

How and When to Use This Sign

→ Sign "Ready" before or after you introduce what's about to happen. For instance, if you're putting your coats on to go outside, sign "Ready."

→ Make an inquisitive facial expression when you ask, "Ready?"

Watch for This!
Your baby may wag their finger back and forth before they learn how to create an *R* letter.

Helping Hand
You can sign "Ready" for nearly every activity with your baby, from running to your car in the rain to going down a slide at the park.

Good Night, Gorilla

SIGNS

• **Goodnight** (p. 96)

How about a bedtime story in sign language? We got you! Rocky Mountain Deaf School has a YouTube channel filled with a library of engaging videos in sign language. Many videos include children's books being read both in sign language and aloud. All you need is a computer or tablet with internet access. For younger babies, you can opt instead to read the books *Good Night, Gorilla* or *Goodnight Moon* (widely available at libraries) and sign "Goodnight" whenever that word appears. Or see step 3 for another "Goodnight" signing option.

1. Do an internet search for "YouTube ASL Good Night Gorilla."

2. As you watch the storyteller sign, sign along with them by signing "Goodnight" each time they sign "Goodnight." Continue to do this every time the storyteller signs "Goodnight." Be ready to sign numerous times at the end of the story when all the animals say "Goodnight" in the zookeeper's bedroom!

3. You can practice this sign by signing "Goodnight" to everything on the way to tucking baby into bed, such as other family members, your pet, and even their favorite plushie.

Note: You might notice a slight difference in how "Banana" is signed in the video compared to how it is taught in this book. Both signs are correct. Many signs have variations, depending on who is signing, where they are from, and their background. These variations are often called "regional signs."

Pictured Signs

~~~~~~~~~~~~~~~~~~~~

SIGNS

- **Good Morning** (p. 94)
- **Goodnight** (p. 96)
- **Bed** (p. 98)
- **Blanket** (p. 102)
- **Toothbrush** (p. 104)

Let's bring this book to life for your baby! For this activity, all you need is a camera, access to a printer, and some tape.

1. Take a picture of the illustrations in this book for the following signs: "Good Morning," "Goodnight," "Bed," "Blanket," and "Toothbrush."

2. Print the pictures in color or black and white.

3. Tape the pictures by the relevant object (such as by the crib for "Good Morning"), where your baby can see it but not touch it.

4. Guide your baby by pointing to a picture, asking what the sign is, and then doing the sign.

5. When they're able to express the sign in the picture, ask them to sign what's in the picture. For example, when your baby wakes up in the morning, you can wave at them with a big smile, then point to the nearby picture that shows the sign for "Good Morning," and ask your baby what the sign is.

6. They may or may not sign back to you. It's okay if you want to show them the sign. Over time, they will pick up on the sign.

Bathing and Getting Ready

Even though babies do great with routines, they like some routine activities better than others. Some babies dislike having their diaper changed and won't lie still. Some babies love bath time and may splash water everywhere. Either way, with sign language, you can let your baby know it's time for a bath or that it's time to change their diaper. This way, if they love bath time, they can excitedly anticipate playing in the water with their duck. Or they can feel informed that they are about to have their diaper changed.

Towel

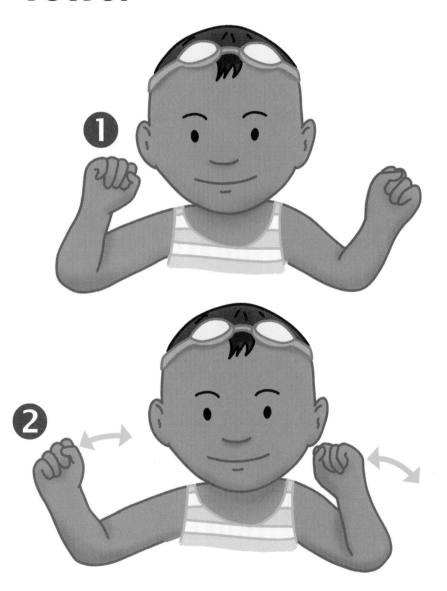

1 With both hands, create fists. Place each fist beside each ear, above the shoulders but not touching your head. **2** Rock your fists side to side, with one fist going toward your ear while the other goes outward, away from your head, and then vice versa. Move your hands back and forth a few times.

How and When to Use This Sign

→ After you give your baby a bath, sign "Towel."

→ You can also sign "Ready" (page 106) after you sign "Towel" to ask your baby if they are ready to get out of the bathtub.

Memory Hack
The sign for a towel is much like the action of rubbing your neck dry with a towel.

Helping Hand
Show your baby how to sign "Towel" by rubbing your neck with a towel. Sign "Towel" again without the towel to show that the action is the same.

Diaper

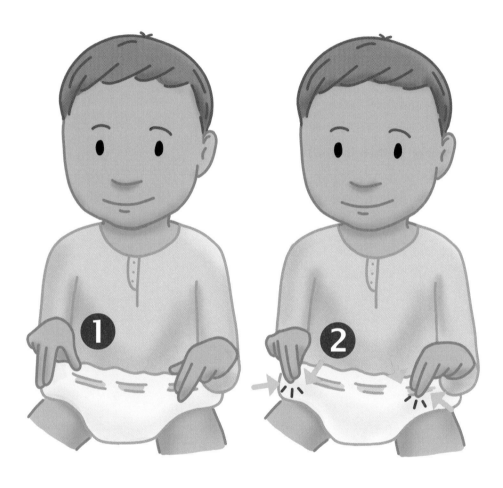

1 With both hands, stick out your index and middle fingers, touching side by side. Stick out your thumbs until they are hovering beneath your middle and index fingers. Bring these handshapes to the front of either side of your hips, one handshape on each side, with fingertips facing down and the thumb closest to the hips. **2** Tap your middle and index fingers against your thumb a couple of times.

How and When to Use This Sign

→ Before you lay your baby down for a diaper change, sign "Diaper."

→ You can also repeat the sign for "Diaper" while simultaneously making a stinky face about their dirty diaper. Once you've put a clean diaper on them, sign "Diaper" again while simultaneously making a happy face.

Memory Hack
The sign for "Diaper" is like placing old-fashioned diaper pins on the front sides of the diaper.

Watch for This!
Your baby may tap their hands onto their hips to sign "Diaper" if they need a change.

Change

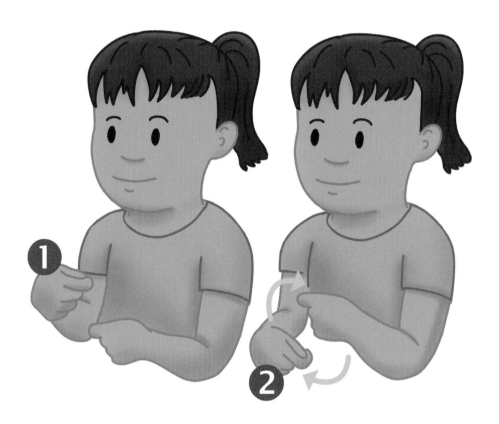

Learn to Sign with Your Baby

1 With both hands, form relaxed fists, bending the index fingers halfway. Have your thumbs touching the bent index fingers. Hold your handshapes in front of your chest, thumb-side up. Hover your dominant handshape directly above the nondominant handshape.

2 Do a half-circle motion with the dominant handshape, moving inward toward your chest and down while the nondominant handshape moves outward and up, until your hands have switched places.

How and When to Use This Sign

→ When you lay your baby down to change them, sign "Change."

→ You can sign "Diaper" before signing "Change" if you are changing their diaper.

Watch for This!
Make sure your hands don't touch when doing the rotation motion or you'll be signing a different word.

Have Fun!
Sign "Change" when you're changing your clothes. You can ask your baby to help you change by picking out an outfit for you. Hold up two shirts and see which they choose for you. Then let them choose an outfit for themself!

Clothes

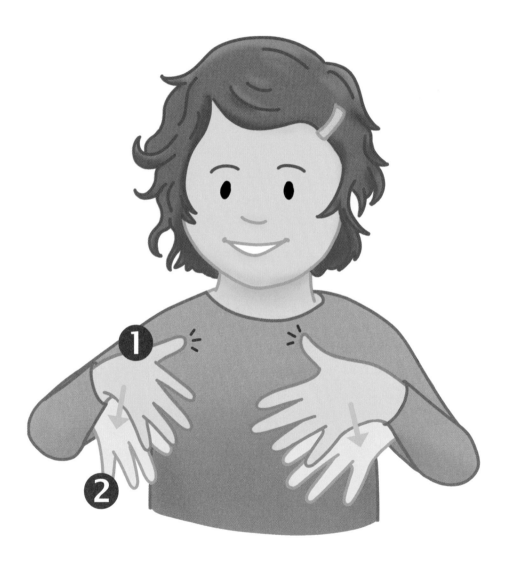

Learn to Sign with Your Baby

1 With both hands, spread out all five fingers. With palms facing your chest, touch the top part of your chest with the inside tips of your thumbs. **2** Brush your thumbs against your chest with a slight one-inch downward motion. Repeat this motion quickly one time.

How and When to Use This Sign

→ Before you help your baby dress, sign "Clothes" to indicate that you are changing their clothes or putting on more layers, like a jacket.

→ You can sign "Change" after signing "Clothes" to communicate that you are changing their clothes. You can sign "Night," as taught in the second part of "Goodnight" (page 96), and then sign "Clothes" to indicate pajamas.

Watch for This!
Your baby may slide their open palms against their chest rather than doing the brushing motion for "Clothes."

Have Fun!
Play dress-up with your baby's doll or stuffed animals and sign "Clothes" while doing this activity. If they can, let them choose the clothes!

Bath

1

2

1 With both hands, form relaxed fists. Stick your thumbs up. **2** With the fingers facing your chest, touch your upper chest. Rub your hands up and down slightly a few times.

How and When to Use This Sign

→ Before you take your baby for a bath, sign "Bath." You can also sign "Bath" while you're filling the tub or sink with water.

→ When you're ready to take your baby from the tub, you can sign "Bath" then "All Done" (page 32).

Memory Hack
The sign for "Bath" is much like the action of scrubbing your chest.

Watch for This!
Like many other signs that require two hands, you may see your baby sign "Bath" with only one hand.

Soap

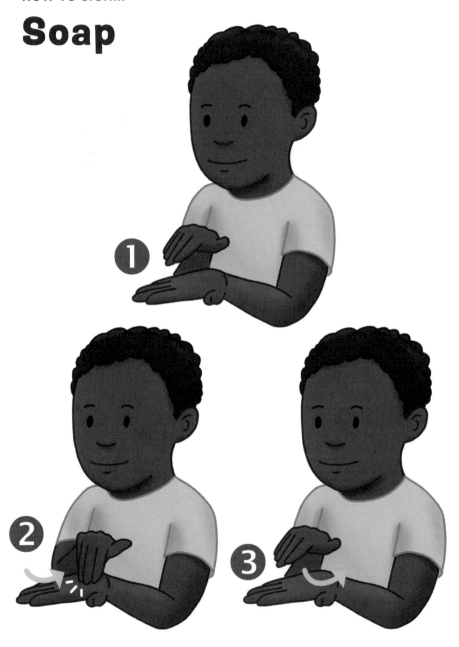

① With your nondominant hand, straighten all fingers, touching except for the thumb. Place this hand in front of your chest comfortably, palm facing up. Create a 90-degree angle with your dominant hand. **②** Brush the inside fingertips of your four dominant fingers in the middle of your nondominant hand's open palm. **③** Repeat the motion a couple of times.

How and When to Use This Sign

→ Before you wash your baby with soap, sign "Soap."

→ Try putting the soap in the palm of your nondominant hand and sign "Soap" with your other hand to associate the sign with the object.

Memory Hack
The sign for "Soap" is much like the action of rubbing a few fingers on a soap bar that you're holding with your other hand.

Helping Hand
Many parents use the sign for "Soap" during bath time, but you can also use it when you wash your hands in the bathroom or before a meal.

Water

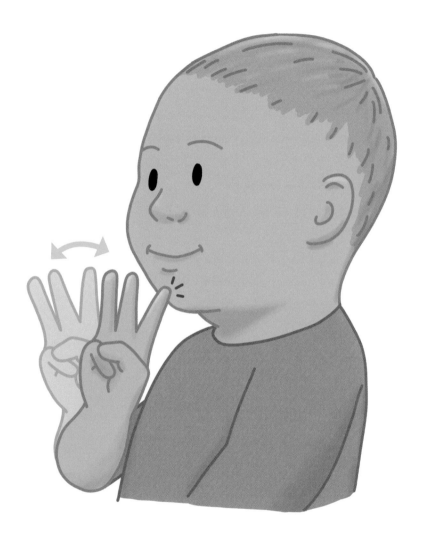

With your dominant hand, straighten out your three middle fingers and spread them out, forming a W shape. Touch the fingertips of your thumb and pinkie together. Bring this handshape to the front of your chin. With the side of your index finger, tap your chin a couple of times.

How and When to Use This Sign

→ Sign "Water" before you place your baby in the water, pour water on their body, or playfully splash the water around them.

→ Sign "Ready" (page 106) with an inquisitive look before signing "Water" to ask your baby if they are ready to go into the water.

Watch for This!
Only tap your chin with the side of your index finger, not with all three middle fingers.

Have Fun!
There are so many fun activities to do with water. You can sign "Water" whenever you interact with water, such as when you swim or do sensory play with water in a bin, or even when you see a body of water.

Duck

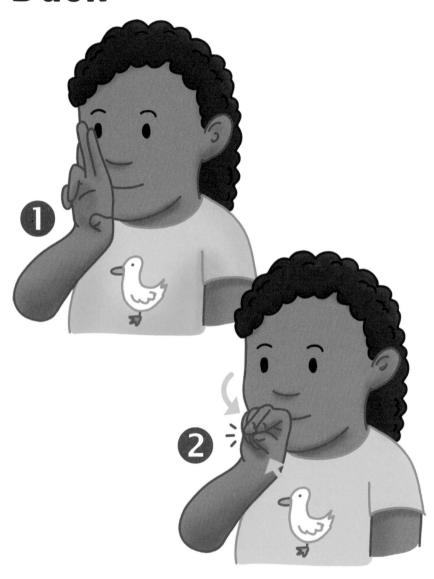

1 With your dominant hand, stick out your index and middle fingers, touching. Stick out your thumb until it's hovering beneath your middle and index fingers. Bring this hand-shape to your mouth, with the outside of your hand near your wrist touching your lips, fingers facing out. **2** Lift up the index and middle fingers, away from the thumb, and then back down until touching your thumb again. Repeat the sign quickly.

How and When to Use This Sign

→ Sign "Duck" when you hand your baby a rubber duck. You can sign "Duck" multiple times while baby plays with their duck.

→ You can sign "Soap" before "Duck" if you are washing their duck, too. You can also sign "Water" before signing "Duck" if you are rinsing the duck with water.

Memory Hack

The sign for "Duck" is like a duck's beak opening and closing.

Watch for This!

If you sign the motion for "Duck" with only one finger (index finger) and thumb, you are signing "Bird." Now there's some bonus material!

ACTIVITY

Bath Count

~~~~~~~~~~

SIGNS

- **Bath** (p. 120)
- **Water** (p. 124)
- **Soap** (p. 122)
- **All Done** (p. 32)
- **Towel** (p. 112)

Let's count our way through some of the signs in this chapter during your baby's bath time! No supplies are needed except for a towel, their duck, and their bath-time products.

1.   When it's time for a bath, hold up one index finger, then sign "Bath."

2.   Right before you place your baby in the water, hold up two fingers (index, middle), then sign "Water."

3.   Once they are wet and you're ready to wash them with soap, hold up three digits (thumb and index and middle fingers), then sign "Soap."

4.   After you wash them with soap, hold up four fingers (index, middle, ring, pinkie), then sign "Water," indicating that you're about to rinse the soap off.

5.   When you're done rinsing them, put up five fingers (all five, including thumb!), then sign "All Done" and "Towel."

Note: This counting activity helps communicate numbers as well as the words/signs you use around bath time. Also, with repetition of this activity, your baby will become familiar with what happens during bath time. Eventually, they may begin to hold up one or more fingers, showing that they are trying to count with you.

Diaper, Diaper

SIGNS

- **Change** (p. 116)
- **Diaper** (p. 114)
- **Clothes** (p. 118)

In this activity, you'll create a routine around diaper changing that is more interactive and fun for your baby than just lying there, exposed and chilly! You don't need anything other than diapering supplies. You'll sign with your body, facial expressions, and hands in a visually rhythmic tone. As your baby grows familiar with it, they may respond to your uplifting movements and sign with facial or bodily enthusiasm. It can go something like this:

1. Before you take off your baby's clothes, sign "Change" as you sway to one side, and then sign "Change" again as you sway back to the other side. Express happiness with this simple dance and acknowledge your baby excitedly as you sign. Try to find your rhythm as you do this with the sign "Change."

2. When you take your baby's clothes off and before you remove their dirty diaper, do the same rhythmic dance, but instead of signing "Change," sign "Diaper."

3. When it's time to put your baby's clothes back on, do the rhythmic dance again as you sign "Clothes."

CHAPTER 7

Playing and Going Out

Playtime is a fun time with your baby. Let's make it the best time with sign language! You can teach your baby how to sign whether they'd like to go on a walk, play with a ball, or read a book. The signs included in this chapter share a mix of getting ready to go outside, a few playtime activities, and some verbs that are useful to communicate what's happening. Be sure to circle back to signs like "My Turn/Your Turn" (page 44), "Where" (page 38), and "Another" (page 42) to enhance your conversation while playing. You can use these signs while taking turns with a toy, asking where to go on a walk, or fetching another ball to play with.

Play

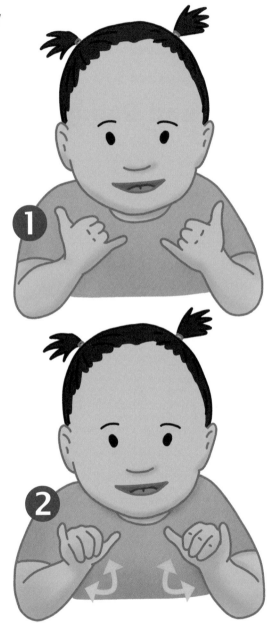

❶ Extend the thumb and pinkie of both hands while the middle three fingers are bent into your palm. **❷** In front of your chest, twist your wrists back and forth a few times.

How and When to Use This Sign

→ Before going outside to play or entering your baby's play space, sign "Play." You can also point to or show what object the baby can play with and sign "Play."

→ You can sign "Ball" (page 142) followed by "Play" to suggest playing with a ball.

Watch for This!
Make sure only your pinkie and thumb are sticking out when you sign "Play."

Have Fun!
While waiting in the doctor's office, sign "Play" before giving your baby choices of toys to play with. For instance, before holding up a baby rattle and a teether toy, sign "Play" to see which one they choose.

Let's Go

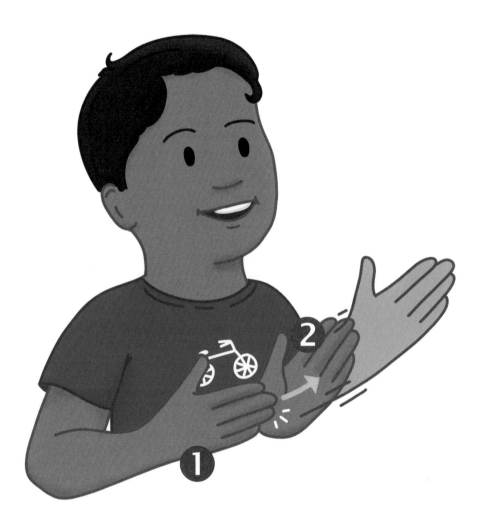

1 With both hands, straighten out all fingers, touching, except for the thumb. In front of your chest, hover both palms facing one another, about an inch apart with your fingers pointing forward. **2** Swiftly brush your dominant palm forward against the nondominant palm, then along your fingers, until the hands are not touching anymore. This motion can be done in a tilted form or slightly sideways, too. (Like several other signs in this book, there are variations to this sign.)

How and When to Use This Sign

→ Right before you're heading out somewhere, sign "Let's Go."

→ To indicate which direction you're suggesting, sign "Let's Go" in movement toward that door or space.

Watch for This!
Make sure you only do a forward, sliding motion of your dominant hand toward the direction you plan to exit.

Helping Hand
To help your baby recognize the motion of signing "Let's Go," you can clap your hands together, wait a moment, and then do the forward, sliding motion of the dominant hand.

Shoes

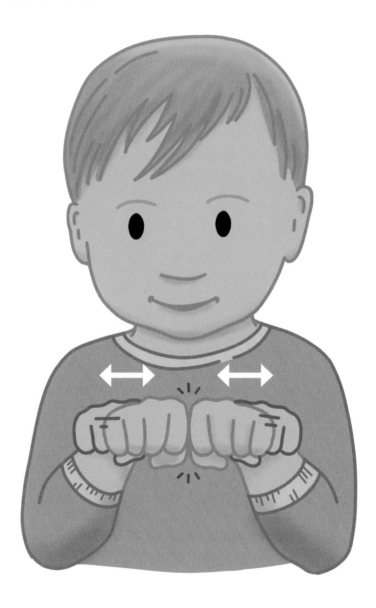

With both hands, create fists, wrapping your thumb around your fingers on each hand. In front of your chest, with the finger-side of your fists facing down, knock your fists together a couple of times.

How and When to Use This Sign

→ Right before you help your baby put their shoes on, sign "Shoes." When you've put on one shoe, sign "Shoes" again before you put on the second one.

→ You can sign "Shoes" followed by "Help" (page 40) to indicate that you will help your baby put their shoes on.

Memory Hack

The motion of signing "Shoes" is much like the action of clacking one's shoes against each other.

Watch for This!

Your baby may not always sign "Shoes" with closed fists with both hands. You may see them sign one hand with a closed fist and the other in a semiclosed fist or even an open hand.

Walk

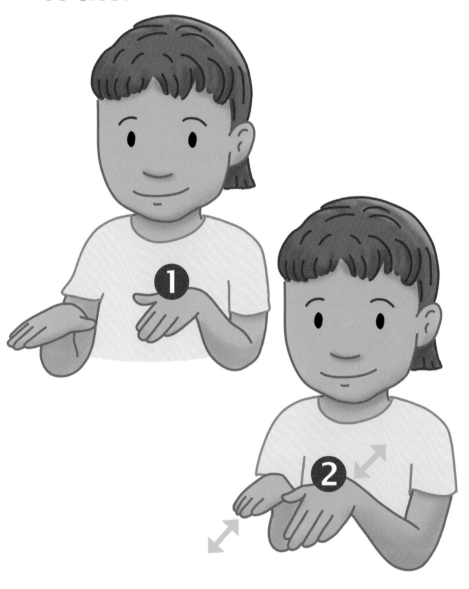

Learn to Sign with Your Baby

① With both hands, straighten your fingers with all fingers touching, except for the thumb. Put these handshapes in front of your chest, palms down. **②** Swing both hands back and forth a couple of times, with the hands going in alternating directions.

How and When to Use This Sign

→ Before you head out the door for a walk, sign "Walk." While you're on your walk, sign "Walk" to communicate what you are doing together.

→ You can sign "Walk" followed by "Let's Go" (page 134) before you head out for a walk.

Memory Hack
The motion for signing "Walk" is much like the action of two feet walking.

Watch for This!
Make sure you do a gentle swinging motion rather than a sliding motion. The sliding motion would be more suitable to describe rollerblading.

Book

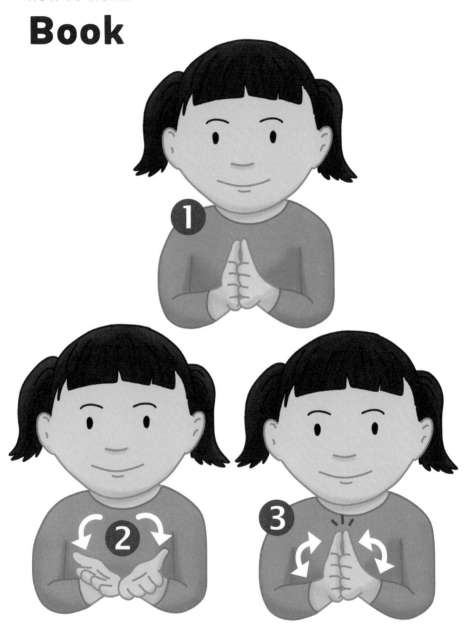

1 With both hands, straighten your fingers with all fingers touching, except for the thumb. Press the insides of your palms together in front of your chest. **2** Twist your wrists so the thumbs turn outward, while keeping the pinkies touching. **3** Close and open your hands again.

How and When to Use This Sign

→ Before you open a book, sign "Book."

→ You can use the sign for "Another" (page 42) to read another book, or sign "All Done" (page 32) when you're done reading a book.

Memory Hack

The sign for a book is much like the action of opening a book.

Have Fun!

Make a book using cardboard for pages (like a board book for babies), and glue pictures of items to the pages, such as duck, ball, apple, bottle, and shoes. Attach the pages to each other with string. Practice signing together with baby's new board book!

Ball

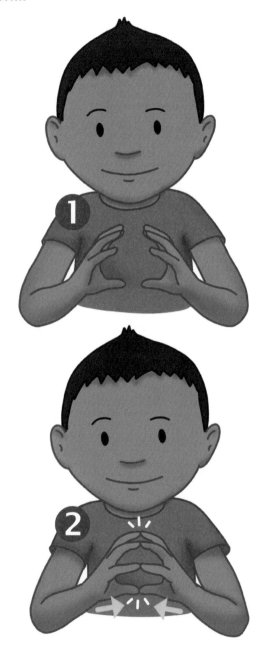

1 With both hands, bend all fingers including the thumb slightly inward as though you're gripping a doorknob, keeping your fingers spread out. **2** In front of your chest, tap the tips of your fingers against their identical fingers on the other hand a couple of times. If you're playing with a bigger ball, your fingertips do not need to touch.

How and When to Use This Sign

→ When you toss or hand a ball over to your baby or you want them to find the ball, sign "Ball."

→ With a ball the size of your palm or smaller, you can sign "Ball" while holding the ball with one hand.

Memory Hack

The sign for "Ball" is similar to hugging both hands on opposite sides of a ball.

Have Fun!

If you attend a sporting event that includes a ball (such as soccer or tennis), talk about the game by pointing where the ball is and signing "Ball." You can also ask your baby to find it by using the signs for "Where" (page 38) and "Ball."

Look

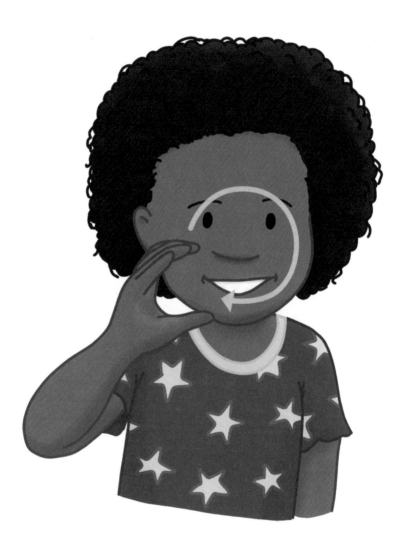

There are a few signs that fit the English word "look." This sign for "Look" indicates you're searching for something. With your dominant hand, create a C shape. Hover the C shape in front of your nose and make mini circular motions a couple of times in front of your nose.

How and When to Use This Sign

→ When you want to search for a misplaced toy, sign "Look" while showing that you're looking around.

→ You can sign "Where" (and state what you're looking for if it's not an object whose sign is taught in this book) followed by "Look."

Watch for This!
Your baby may sign "Look" with a circular motion in front of their face but may not use the right handshape.

Have Fun!
Use this sign for games such as looking for pets or wild animals on your walk, seashells on the beach, or rocks on a hike.

Paying Signs Forward

SIGNS

- **Shoes** (p. 136)
- **Let's Go** (p. 134)
- **Walk** (p. 138)
- **Look** (p. 144)
- **Ball** (p. 142)
- **Play** (p. 132)

This activity presents a great opportunity to share signs you've learned with your baby. You can share any of the signs in this chapter—or in this book—whenever you're out or when someone visits.

1. Let's say you and your visitor decide to go outside for a walk together. Show your visitor the sign for "Shoes," "Let's Go," and "Walk."

2. As you walk, explain and demonstrate "Look" as you look for certain things. While outside, look for opportunities to use signs like "Ball" and "Play."

3. While you "pay it forward" with these signs, allow your baby to observe this other person using the same signs they know.

Hide-and-Seek

SIGNS

- **Play** (p. 132)
- **Look** (p. 144)

Every child enjoys a classic game of hide-and-seek, right? Let's get some signing involved while you're at it! All you need to know are the signs for "Play" and "Look." You'll see two variations of this game: one for young children who can hide and one for babies who aren't mobile yet.

1. Sign "Play" and then tell your child to go hide and that you'll look for them by signing "Look." Even if your child just hides under a blanket in front of you, you definitely can play along with that idea of hiding, too.

2. Keep signing "Look" in case they're peeking through a crack or around the corner.

3. If your baby isn't mobile yet, you can also play this while hiding a plushie. Sign "Play," then cover their plushie with a blanket. Sign "Look," look around like you forgot where you put it, and finally, uncover!

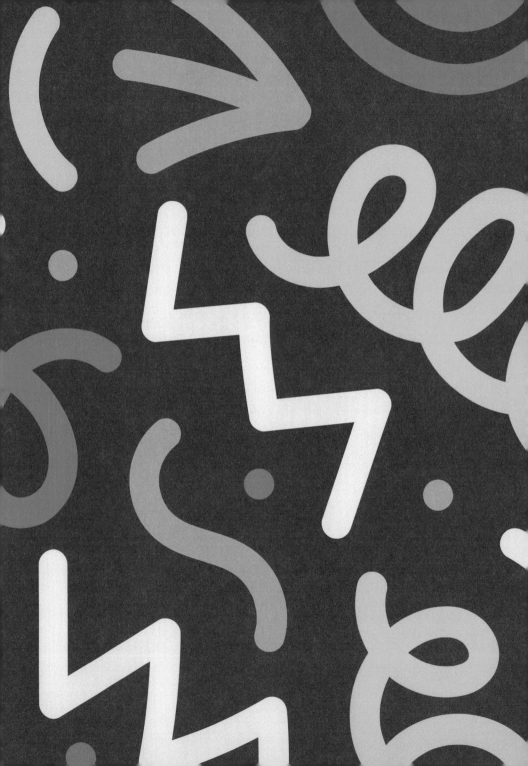

Conclusion

Wow! You've done it! You've learned at least 50 signs to communicate with your baby. While it takes practice, time, and a bit of persistence until your baby understands and expresses all 50 signs, you've done the most important part by learning them and testing them out. Keep on using them; you have a wealthy bank of essential signs to communicate with your baby, and they'll catch on in time.

Keep this book nearby in case you need a refresher. It's okay if you forget how to do a sign; that's what this book is here for. This book can also come in handy if you want to expand your knowledge after learning all 50 signs—just check out the resources section on page 150. If you want to continue your journey with learning and using ASL with your child beyond this book, you could also take a beginner ASL course offered by Deaf instructors. Check out social media—there are many wonderful Deaf teachers who teach signs for free.

One final activity: Your baby ought to know how loved they are, considering your commitment to this wonderful endeavor with them. If you haven't yet had the chance today, tell your baby you love them by signing "I Love You."

Next, ask them for a hug, because you both have been awesome at this!

Finally, close this book and have at it!

Resources

LEARN ASL

Learn to Sign with Your Baby
Video Supplements
To help you visualize and practice
the signs from the previous chapters,
use the following QR code to access
videos of all the signs contained in
this book, or visit signwithyourbaby.
zeitgeistpublishing.com.

The ASL App
theaslapp.com
Phone app that offers 2,500+ con-
versational signs and phrases in
American Sign Language

ASL Connect
gallaudet.edu/asl-connect
Introductory videos and interactive les-
sons to learn American Sign Language,
along with five levels of ASL courses and
10+ diverse course materials for ASL

ASL University
lifeprint.com
Sign language library and enrichment
for students, teachers, interpreters,
and parents

Dawn Sign Press
dawnsign.com
Videos that teach American Sign
Language, including signed fairy tales

**The Gallaudet Children's Dictionary
of American Sign Language**
gcdasl.com
A book of drawings and online videos
teaching 1,000+ signs

RMDSCO
youtube.com/user/RMDSCO
YouTube channel curated by Rocky
Mountain Deaf School, filled with a
library of engaging videos in sign
language

Sign Language Center
signlanguagecenter.com
Online and in-person American Sign
Language courses, workshops, and
tutoring

OTHER RESOURCES

American Sign Language at Home
aslathome.org
Website providing a family-centered curriculum for families with young deaf children and the professionals who support them. While this curriculum is primarily designed for deaf children, it can also be applied to hearing children using ASL at home.

The Ariel Series
thearielseries.com
Author and their family's journey in using ASL. Follow them on Instagram, TikTok, and Twitter @thearielseries.

"Bilingualism in the Early Years: What the Science Says" by Krista Byers-Heinlein and Casey Lew-Williams
ncbi.nlm.nih.gov/pmc/articles/ PMC6168212
Article presenting research that suggests that early bilingual development enhances a child's language development and acquisition

California Department of Education: Language Development Milestones
cde.ca.gov/sp/ss/dh/sb210langmile stones.asp
Website providing information about sign language milestones in a child's development

"Enhancing Early Communication through Infant Sign Training" by Rachel H. Thompson, Nicole M. Cotnoir-Bichelman, Paige M. McKerchar, Trista L. Tate, and Kelly A. Dancho
ncbi.nlm.nih.gov/pmc/articles/ PMC1868823
Article presenting research that suggests benefits to using sign language with hearing babies who have not yet developed the ability to verbally communicate

"The Role of Sign Language in Overcoming Learning Disability for Children" by Samplius
samplius.com/free-essay-examples/ the-role-of-sign-language-in-overcoming-learning-disability-for-children
Essay supporting the idea that use of sign language with children who may have a learning disability may help bridge a gap in communication

West Virginia Department of Education: Office of Special Education
wvde.state.wv.us/osp/
ASLDevelopmentalchecklist.pdf
Document providing a consolidation of multisource information regarding American Sign Language development in babies and children

IDEAL American Sign Language and English Language Development Milestones
in.gov/health/cdhhe/files/ideal-
language-milestones-english-
american-sign-language.pdf
Document providing language milestones for American Sign Language and English from newborns to 11-year-olds

VCSL Visual Communication and Sign Language Checklist by Simms, Baker, & Clark, 2013
gallaudet.edu/clerc-center-sites/
Documents/Clerc%20Microsite/
Assets/Simms_Baker_Clark-VCSL-
SLS-2013.pdf
Document providing sign language milestones in a checklist format from birth to five-year-olds

ASL Stages of Development, Early Childhood Education Department, California School for the Deaf
successforkidswithhearingloss.com/
wp-content/uploads/2011/12/ASL-
Stages-of-Development-Assmt.pdf
Document providing listed ASL stages of development from three-month-olds to six-year-olds

Index

Entries for the 50 essential signs are listed in **boldface**.

About the Author

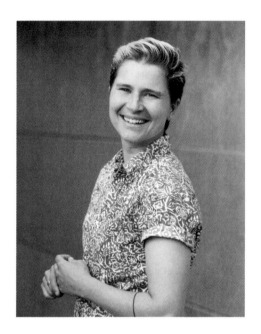

Cecilia (C3) Grugan is a Deaf parent to a hearing child, who is referred to as a Child of Deaf Adults (CODA). Cecilia lives in the suburbs of Washington, DC, with their partner, who is also Deaf, and firstborn. As a family, they solely use American Sign Language (ASL). With ASL, Grugan's family thrives on access and ease of communication with one another. When not writing during the darkest hour, Cecilia can be found jogging with a stroller around town, exploring new local joints with their partner, or jet-setting across the country in pursuit of new adventures with their firstborn.

Find more about the author at thearielseries.com and follow them on Instagram, TikTok, and Twitter @thearielseries.

About the Illustrator

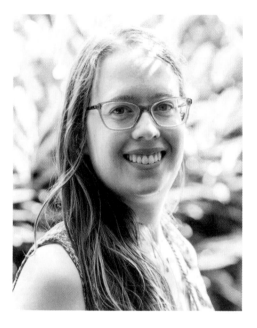

Brittany Castle is a Deaf graphic artist and the owner of 58 Creativity, where she creates and sells American Sign Language art and products. She grew up in California with her Deaf twin sister and their hearing parents. After graduating from Gallaudet University, she began working as a freelance graphic designer but quickly discovered her passion for creating her own art infused with Deaf culture. In 2014 she founded 58 Creativity and has been running it ever since.

Find out more about Brittany at 58creativity.com and follow her on Instagram and Facebook @58Creativity.

Hi there,

We hope you enjoyed *Learn to Sign with Your Baby*. If you have any questions or concerns about your book, or have received a damaged copy, please contact **customerservice@penguinrandomhouse.com**. We're here and happy to help.

Also, please consider writing a review on your favorite retailer's website to let others know what you thought of the book!

Sincerely,

The Zeitgeist Team